Trauma-Informed and Trauma-Responsive Yoga Teaching

of related interest

Trauma-Informed Yoga for Pain Management
A Practical Manual for Simple Stretching, Gentle Strengthening, and Mindful Breathing
Yael Calhoun with Mona Bingham
ISBN 978 1 83997 800 5
eISBN 978 1 83997 801 2

Yoga Therapy for Children and Teens with Complex Needs
A Somatosensory Approach to Mental, Emotional and Physical Wellbeing
Shawnee Thornton Hardy
Foreword by Amy Wheeler
ISBN 978 1 78775 225 2
eISBN 978 1 78775 226 9

Yoga of Recovery
Integrating Yoga and Ayurveda with Modern Recovery Tools for Addiction
Durga Leela
Foreword by David Frawley
ISBN 978 1 78775 755 4
eISBN 978 1 78775 756 1

Transforming Ethnic and Race-Based Traumatic Stress with Yoga
Gail Parker
Illustrations by Justine Ross
ISBN 978 1 78775 753 0
eISBN 978 1 78775 754 7

Trauma-Informed and Trauma-Responsive YOGA TEACHING

A UNIVERSAL PRACTICE

**Catherine Cook-Cottone
and Joanne Spence**

Forewords by Dr. Shirley Telles and Dr. Gail Parker

Illustrations by Masha Pimas

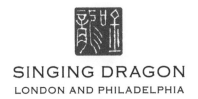

SINGING DRAGON
LONDON AND PHILADELPHIA

First published in Great Britain in 2024 by Singing Dragon,
an imprint of Jessica Kingsley Publishers
Part of John Murray Press

1

Copyright © Catherine Cook-Cottone and Joanne Spence 2024
Illustrations copyright © Masha Pimas 2024
Foreword copyright © Dr. Shirley Telles 2024
Foreword copyright © Dr. Gail Parker 2024

The right of Catherine Cook-Cottone and Joanne Spence to be identified as the Author of the Work has been asserted by them in accordance with the Copyright, Designs and Patents Act 1988.

Front cover image source: VectorStock

All rights reserved. No part of this publication may be reproduced, stored in a retrieval system, or transmitted, in any form or by any means without the prior written permission of the publisher, nor be otherwise circulated in any form of binding or cover other than that in which it is published and without a similar condition being imposed on the subsequent purchaser.

A CIP catalogue record for this title is available from the
British Library and the Library of Congress

ISBN 978 1 83997 816 6
eISBN 978 1 83997 817 3

Printed and bound in the United States by Integrated Books International

Jessica Kingsley Publishers' policy is to use papers that are natural, renewable and recyclable products and made from wood grown in sustainable forests. The logging and manufacturing processes are expected to conform to the environmental regulations of the country of origin.

Singing Dragon
Carmelite House
50 Victoria Embankment
London EC4Y 0DZ

www.singingdragon.com

John Murray Press
Part of Hodder & Stoughton Limited
An Hachette UK Company

Dedication

CATHERINE COOK-COTTONE

*To my family Jerry, Chloe, Maya, and Stephen
and to the yoga students and clients who will always be my greatest teachers*

JOANNE SPENCE

To my beloveds: Doug, Merryn, Jacob, and Lucca

Contents

Foreword by Dr. Shirley Telles 9

Foreword by Dr. Gail Parker 11

Acknowledgments 14

List of Trauma-Informed and Responsive (TIR) Principles for Teaching Yoga 16

List of Trauma-Informed and Responsive (TIR) Practices 24

Introduction 28

Part I: Foundations of Trauma-Informed and Responsive Yoga Teaching

1. Trauma-Informed and Responsive Methods Defined 39
2. Trauma Basics and Terminology 50
3. Preparedness—Resource, Assess, Pause, De-escalate, and Connect 65
4. Mindful Self-Care as a Trauma-Informed and Responsive Practice 78

Part II: Research and Theory: Embodiment, Polyvagal Theory, and Sensations

5. Positive Embodiment, Interoception, and Self-Regulation 99
6. Polyvagal Theory, Window of Tolerance, and Co-Regulation . . . 109
7. Sensations—The Basics 127

8. Sensations as Communication—Physiology, Emotions, Memories, and State Activation 135

9. Sensations and Self-Regulation. 145

Part III: Trauma-Informed and Responsive Communication

10. Communication Basics—Mindful and Heartful Listening 155

11. Nonviolent Communication and Conflict 160

12. Content Warnings, Microaggressions, and Inclusive Language . . 170

13. Trauma-Informed and Responsive Cueing and Assisting. 182

Part IV: Trauma-Informed and Responsive Yoga Teaching Practices

14. Teaching Self-Awareness and Attunement—Being With and Working With 203

15. Practices that Soothe and Calm 218

16. Practices that Activate and Stimulate 237

17. Practices that Balance and Integrate. 255

18. Cultivating a Trauma-Informed and Responsive Yoga Space. . . . 273

References 287

Index 294

Foreword by Dr. Shirley Telles

As part of our school days, most of us would remember teachers whose classes were enjoyable and instructive, whereas others were not as enjoyable and may even have led to a lifelong distaste for a particular area of study. This is true for yoga as well. Studying yoga is a very distinctive, personal, and experiential journey, closely related to most aspects of an individual's life and functioning. A yoga instructor can add considerable depth and value to a yoga student's experience. However, sometimes sincere and entirely well-intentioned yoga teachers may inadvertently infringe on their yoga students' sense of comfort and safety.

All yoga teachers can benefit from verifying that their teaching methods are in tune with the principles of yoga and requirements of a yoga seeker. In short, they are "trauma-informed." Being "trauma-informed" would mean integrating the science and theory of trauma with the principles of yoga, likely to create a harmonious and positive experience of yoga and least likely to intimidate a yoga seeker.

Trauma-Informed and Trauma-Responsive Yoga Teaching: A Universal Practice is *not* a book on yoga to heal trauma (though yoga therapists working with trauma healing would definitely benefit from the knowledge); instead, it is a book intended for every yoga teacher, to understand how to create a safe and nurturing space for yoga instruction based on contemporary knowledge of physiology and yoga tradition.

The authors are certified yoga instructors and recognized yoga therapists. Catherine Cook-Cottone, with a doctorate in psychology, and Joanne Spence, with a master's in theology, take the reader on a journey to discover, understand, and practice trauma-informed yoga in easy stages. Beginning with an introduction to concepts relevant to both trauma and yoga, the early chapters cover empowering concepts such as positive embodiment, "neuroception" (Stephen Porges' term for the ability to assess safety and threat), and self-regulation. The polyvagal theory is presented with clarity and simplicity, while explaining the application of the theory as the authors discuss the importance of communication to create the desired space for the yoga experience. Other interesting points which are covered include the rationale and science underlying practices to soothe and calm, to activate and stimulate, and to balance and integrate ourselves. In keeping with the general sense and purpose of the book, the authors emphasize the importance of honoring the history and practice of yoga, which is relevant to all yoga instructors. Finally, the authors suitably place an emphasis on a yoga instructor's mindful self-care, as an important part of being a worthy teacher of yoga.

I believe that *Trauma-Informed and Trauma-Responsive Yoga Teaching: A Universal Practice* will add value to any yoga instructor's journey, by deepening their knowledge and experience of yoga while they mentor others with sensitivity and spread the ancient wisdom.

Shirley Telles, PhD
Researcher and Director
Patanjali Research Foundation

Foreword by Dr. Gail Parker

I know trauma from personal experience, as a psychotherapist, a yoga therapist educator, and as an author who has written two books about how yoga can ease the pain and suffering of those who have been traumatized. I'd like to share a bit of my personal story with you.

I am what they call a military brat, a term of endearment in military culture that describes children of parents who serve(d) full-time in the United States Armed Forces. My father was one of the original Tuskegee Airmen, the African American pilots who flew hundreds of successful missions as bomber escorts over North Africa and Europe during World War II. The Red-Tail Angels helped destroy Adolf Hitler's regime and defeat Nazi tyranny, at the same time helping to end racial segregation in the United States armed services. After World War II ended, my father went on to make the military his full-time career.

When I was five years old, my mother and I took a train from Detroit, Michigan, to Seattle, Washington, where we boarded a ship bound for Tokyo, Japan, to join my father. He was fighting in the Korean War. Tachikawa Airfield in the western part of Tokyo would be our new home for the duration of his deployment. The trip was stressful! En route to Seattle, our train derailed. Fortunately, no one was injured, but I remember being stranded outside on a cold, snowy night, for how long I don't remember. What I do remember is feeling the security and warmth of my mother's presence. We eventually arrived safely in Seattle where we embarked on the ship that would take us to our new home. It was a three-week journey, and it was rough. My mother said we encountered seven typhoons, which are storms that form over the Pacific Ocean and are equivalent to hurricanes in intensity. All I remember of the trip is how seasick I was for what seemed like forever, and the warmth and reassuring presence of my mother's comfort. When we finally arrived in Tokyo, I remember my father picking me up, holding me close, and hugging me tight. In his embrace, with my mother next to me, I knew that everything was going to be alright. Little did I know.

My mother was only 26 years old at the time and in no way prepared for the realities of living as a military wife and mother of a young child in a foreign country, in a war zone, lonely for friends and family, while also navigating the stress and trauma of racism in a recently desegregated military that she, the Black officers, and their wives and children were exposed to daily. Eventually, the stress became overwhelming, and my mother had what was then called a nervous breakdown. She was misdiagnosed as being mentally ill, hospitalized, medicated, and returned to the United States alone, to be hospitalized in a strange city with no family or friends while she waited for my father, who had been reassigned, to join her. I remained in Japan with my father. It was traumatic for all of us.

To be clear, although my mother was treated as if she was mentally ill, she was not. She was traumatized. Trauma is a specific type of stress that reflects exposure to terrible events generally outside the range of daily human experience that are emotionally painful, intense, and distressing. Back then, trauma-informed approaches to mental health and wellbeing did not exist. The thinking was if you became overwhelmed by stress, it was because you weren't mentally or morally strong or tough enough, that there was something wrong with you. A trauma-informed approach would have considered that it was not my mother's mental health that was the problem, but the accumulation of stressors that overwhelmed her capacity to process the events she experienced.

We are a society embedded in a state of unhealed cumulative trauma. We are traumatized emotionally, physiologically, spiritually, and interpersonally. Even though the effects of stress and trauma abound, many of us remain unaware of its effects because it's so common. Within the past four years, we have endured a deadly global pandemic, an alarming increase in gun violence, domestic violence, open expressions of anti-Black racism, antisemitism, xenophobia, a threat to the bodily autonomy of women, social isolation, loss of community, and more. It has been traumatic.

Trauma disconnects us from ourselves and from each other. Yoga brings us back to self and invites us into community. People are turning to yoga as a self-care modality for stress relief and to ease the distress of trauma. Increasing numbers of first responders, firefighters, law enforcement personnel, and health care providers are turning to yoga practices for relief. Doctors and mental health care providers are recommending yoga as beneficial to their stressed and traumatized patients. As a result, it behooves all yoga teachers and yoga therapists to be trauma-informed because, in all likelihood, there will be someone coming to your yoga class or coming to you for yoga therapy who has been traumatized. Trauma-informed yoga is a practice that can help relieve current suffering and prevent future suffering.

Catherine Cook-Cottone, a licensed psychologist, and Joanne Spence, a self-described "recovering social worker," know this. Both are also certified yoga therapists and authors on trauma-informed yoga. They have written *Trauma-Informed and Trauma-Responsive Yoga Teaching: A Universal Practice*, a timely book that advocates and argues for all yoga teachers and yoga therapists to adopt trauma-informed methods in their teaching. Not all yoga teacher trainings include trauma-informed yoga as part of their curriculum, and even if you have taken trauma-informed yoga teacher training, refining your knowledge is an ongoing process. This book will help you understand what it means to be trauma-informed and offers step-by-step teaching points to guide you. You may never hear the stories of your students, and the authors make it clear that you are not being asked to treat trauma. That is within the purview of licensed professionals. A trauma-informed approach to teaching yoga, they tell us, emphasizes choice, empowerment, and a felt sense of safety in your teaching that allows your students to reconnect to themselves, to one another, and to experience a sense of agency in the process. The authors invite you to examine your own unhealed trauma as part of your journey so you can be more effective in your teaching.

Trauma-Informed and Trauma-Responsive Yoga Teaching: A Universal Practice is a book that offers a common-sense approach to trauma-informed teaching and includes foundational concepts and practical teaching practices, and ends by exploring trauma-informed teaching as a spiritual and professional path. It is comprehensive, easy to read, and should be required reading for all yoga teachers and yoga therapists. I only wish it had been available during my mother's lifetime.

Gail Parker, PhD, C-IAYT
Psychologist, Yoga Therapist Educator, and Author of Restorative Yoga for Ethnic and Race-Based Stress and Trauma *and* Transforming Race-Based Traumatic Stress with Yoga

Acknowledgments

We would like to acknowledge first the transformational role yoga philosophies and practices have had in our lives. Thank you to Sarah Hamlin who believed in the book and helped us bring it to life. Our illustrator, Masha Pimas, took our vision of yoga's inclusive nature and ran with it. We are so pleased with the result.

We'd like to formally thank Dr. Shirley Telles and Dr. Gail Parker for their beautiful forewords: one from a researcher's perspective, and one from a clinician's perspective respectively. We owe a great debt to each of you for the paths you have forged for us and for yoga teachers for decades.

A big thank you to Maya Cottone who carefully edited each page of this book. And to Merryn Spence for critiquing each chapter from her lens as an early adopter of trauma-informed and trauma-responsive yoga teaching. Thank you also to Calry Pershyn for your thoughtful feedback.

I (CCC) would like to acknowledge the university students, clients, and yoga students who have practiced and studied with me to co-create my understanding of these practices. I can only truly come to know things through my embodied experiences – a process which is a deeply social act. Each yoga class, yoga session, and university lecture and discussion teaches me, and we all grow. This co-created learning is woven into every page of this book. In this way, each of my students and clients is a co-author of these pages. Thank you. A quick thank you to Finnegan, Hobbes, Taffy, Soka, and Willow, who all happily nestled into my writing room with me, making it a warm and productive place to be. I am also deeply grateful to Joanne, who lives these practices and reminds me that yoga is not just for the yoga mat; it is for meetings about book deadlines, lively debates in backyards, and for the work of being the kindest and most thoughtful versions of ourselves. Thank you, Joanne, for bringing these practices to life on the pages of this book, through your work with our illustrator, Masha Pimas, the sharing of your yoga teaching trials and tribulations, and for your graceful partnership with me. Last, and perhaps most importantly, I acknowledge and am grateful for the transformative power of yoga in my life.

I (JS) am grateful for feedback from Katrina Woodworth, Eva Trapp, and Allyson Huval. Books often don't get finished without quiet and beautiful places for authors to hide out in. Thank you to Christine and Mark Guy for providing such a place when I needed it the most. Anytime I write about yoga, I am always picturing the many students I have taught over the years as I try to articulate something that I think will be helpful to yoga teachers in training. I have deep gratitude for each of you. I'd like to give a special shout out to my writing people—all 45 or so (including our fearless leader Shan, and our administrative team, Donna, Denise, Jane, Ramona, Drew, our teachers), and 34 cohort members of the inaugural Doctor of Ministry in Creative Writing and Public Theology program at Pittsburgh Theological Seminary. Your encouragement and support have been crucial to my wellbeing during the writing of this book, even when you didn't know it. I am most grateful to Catherine for inviting me into the wild adventure of writing this book with you. I am fortunate to be blessed by your writing skills, your work ethic, and your deep knowledge of the field. But most of all, I have enjoyed your collaborative congeniality and friendship. Writing can be lonely and isolating, but this project certainly was not. Finally, I stand in awe of the ancient practice of yoga that has changed my life for the better. Through this book, you may begin to understand why, and your life will change for the better also.

List of Trauma-Informed and Responsive (TIR) Principles for Teaching Yoga

Chapter 1

- Yoga Is Personal
  Yoga is an intimate practice, through which you develop your own relationship with each of the eight limbs in a way that meets you exactly where you are.

- Choice and Agency
  Experiencing trauma usually involves lack of choice or personal agency; therefore, teaching in a trauma-informed way begins with choice and agency.

- Safety
  Feeling safe is a personal, subjective experience that varies from student to student, minute to minute, pose to pose, and context to context.

Chapter 2

- Trauma and Impact
  Trauma is not defined by the event; it is defined by the impact of the event on the nervous system.

- Traumatic Exposure Varies
  Traumatic exposure varies by intensity, duration, frequency, pace, chronicity, breadth, and complexity.

LIST OF TIR PRINCIPLES FOR TEACHING YOGA

- **Posttraumatic Growth**
  Posttraumatic growth is possible, and yoga can help.

- **Trauma Is Universal**
  Trauma is a universal experience affecting people across cultures, countries, races and ethnicities, incomes, gender identities, and ages.

Chapter 3

- **Develop Inner Resources**
  Encourage the development of inner resources, or internal aids, that you can turn to when you need support.

- **Self-Regulation Scale**
  Use the self-regulation scale to assess your state and the state of your students.

- **Practicing the PAUSE**
  Any time, any place, and for any reason, you can always PAUSE. Pause = stop what you are doing, A = assess how you are and what you need, and USE = use your resources.

- **Sometimes Just Breathing Together Is Enough**
  Intentional, gentle, and slow breathing can help down-regulate a dysregulated nervous system.

- **Know a De-escalation Protocol**
  Yoga teachers should know and be prepared to implement a de-escalation protocol—recognize, stabilize, and refer.

Chapter 4

- **The More You Care, the More You Need Self-Care**
  Those who care the most are at the highest risk for burnout and compassion fatigue. The need for self-care is even higher for those who care a lot.

- **Scope of Practice**
  Teach within your scope of practice.

- **Professional Boundaries**
  Keeping professional boundaries is good for you and your yoga students.

- **Nemo Dat Quod Non Habet**
  You cannot give what you do not have.

- **Practice Is Everything**
  Your personal practice will be the foundation of your trauma-informed yoga teaching.

- **Mindful Self-Care Is a Generous Act**
  Engaging in mindful self-care is something that benefits both you and the people in your life. You become the best version of yourself for you and them.

- **Mindful Self-Care Is Collective Care**
  Your mindful self-care should serve, and not interfere with, others' mindful self-care.

Chapter 5

- **The Issues Are in Our Tissues**
  Trauma memories can be stored in the body as nonverbal, physical sensations in muscles and movement, breath patterns, heart rate, feeling-sensations, and action urges.

- **Neuroception**
  Neuroception is the nervous system's automatic process of evaluating safety and threat without requiring awareness.

- **Orienting for Safety**
  Take a moment before practice to orient for safety.

Chapter 6

- **Polyvagal Theory**
  Take time to know, understand, and apply the polyvagal theory to yourself and your students.

LIST OF TIR PRINCIPLES FOR TEACHING YOGA

- **Connection and Protection**
  Those who have been through trauma are sensitized toward protection over connection.

- **Safe and Uncomfortable**
  Individuals who have experienced trauma sometimes misinterpret the discomfort that comes from growth and learning as feeling unsafe.

- **Great Effort and Great Rest**
  Sustainability is supported by cycling periods of effort and rest. Effort enhances rest and rest supports effort.

- **Practicing the PAUSE**
  Any time, any place, and for any reason, you can always PAUSE. Pause = stop what you are doing, A = assess how you are and what you need, and USE = use your resources.

Chapter 7

- **Sensations Are Communications**
  Our bodies communicate the state of our physiological and emotional selves through sensations.

- **Sensations and Safety**
  There is no universal relationship between safety and sensations that can be applied to all people.

- **Discomfort and Growth**
  Working with discomfort and reactions to it is critical for growth and healing.

Chapter 8

- **Sensations Are Experiences and Communications**
  Sensations are experiences that arise and pass which tell us about our embodied experiences.

- **Practicing the PAUSE**
  Any time, any place, and for any reason, you can always PAUSE. Pause

= stop what you are doing, A = assess how you are and what you need, and USE = use your resources.

Chapter 9
- Meet the Student Exactly Where They Are
  Trauma-informed yoga meets the yoga student exactly where they are with non-judgment, loving-kindness, and carefully scaffolded instruction.

Chapter 10
- Humans Have a Fundamental Need to Be Seen and Heard
  Learn and practice mindful and heartful listening in which seeing and hearing are prioritized over being right and problem solving.

Chapter 11
- Trauma-Informed and Responsive Communication Is Nonviolent
  Learn and practice the principles of nonviolent communication.

- Practicing the PAUSE
  Any time, any place, and for any reason, you can always PAUSE. Pause = stop what you are doing, A = assess how you are and what you need, and USE = use your resources.

Chapter 12
- Use Content Warnings
  Using content warnings lets your students prepare for the content you will be delivering.

- Privacy and Discretion
  Honoring privacy and using discretion in what you share about others honors the trauma-informed values of personal agency and self-determination.

- Trauma-Informed and Responsive Communication Is Inclusive
  Learn and practice using inclusive language.

LIST OF TIR PRINCIPLES FOR TEACHING YOGA

- ▸ Trauma-Informed Yoga Teachers Address Microaggressions
  Be mindful of and address microaggressions as they occur.

Chapter 13

- ▸ Emphasize Intentional, Self-Determined Mobilization and Immobilization
  Yoga is the intentional, self-determined practice of mobilizing and immobilizing the body in service of the body and soul.

- ▸ Offer Practice Making Choices
  "Yoga offers a way to practice making small, manageable choices in relation to one's body" (Emerson & Hopper, 2011, p. 45).

- ▸ Offer Explicit, Ongoing, Informed Consent
  Consent must be clear, continuously given, and based on access to information.

- ▸ Establish the Fundamental Choice to Stop
  To be trauma-informed and responsive, your yoga teaching must create access for your students to the fundamental choice to stop at any point.

- ▸ Be Mindful of Appeasement (or Fawning)
  Yoga students may engage in appeasement when they perceive a power differential, are seeking acceptance, and/or feel threatened.

- ▸ Offer Options
  To make an informed, empowered choice, students need information about ways to accommodate, modify, or expand the pose.

Chapter 14

- ▸ Being with Can Be Transformational
  Being with sensations in the present moment can be a transformational experience.

- ▸ Practicing the PAUSE
  Any time, any place, and for any reason, you can always PAUSE. Pause = stop what you are doing, A = assess how you are and what you need, and USE = use your resources.

- **Highlight Breath in Each and Every Class**
  Set a firm intention to highlight the breath in each and every yoga class you teach.

- **Develop Skills to Be with Emotions**
  Help students develop skills for being with their emotions and associated sensations.

- **Trauma and State Activation Can Shape Thoughts**
  Invite students to notice, name, and reorient their thinking patterns.

- **Teach Attunement**
  Teach to noticing sensations, being with what is there, and intentionally choosing being with or working with based on what is noticed.

Chapter 15

- **Practice in Your Pain-Free Range of Motion**
  Encourage students to move within their pain-free range of motion (staying within the comfort and growth zones).

- **Connect Breath to Movement**
  Encourage students to connect breath to movement.

- **Practicing the PAUSE**
  Any time, any place, and for any reason, you can always PAUSE. Pause = stop what you are doing, A = assess how you are and what you need, and USE = use your resources.

Chapter 18

- **You Cannot Promise a Safe Space**
  Offering a safe space is not possible. Feeling safe is a subjective experience and, as such, cannot be assured.

- **TIR Yoga Teachers Self-Regulate**
  Take time to self-regulate as part of your personal and pre-teaching practices.

LIST OF TIR PRINCIPLES FOR TEACHING YOGA

- **Cultivate Communities of Care**
  TIR communities are continuously developing and evolving communities of care.

- **Yoga Offers Guidance**
  TIR communities study and practice the Yamas and Niyamas.

- **Create Community Agreements**
  Community agreements can support TIR practices.

- **Offer Yoga as a Spiritual and Secular Practice**
  TIR yoga honors the spirituality of yoga while providing practices that are welcoming to all.

- **Trauma-Informed and Responsive Spaces Are Unique**
  TIR spaces are developed and maintained to meet the unique histories, needs, and preferences of the community.

List of Trauma-Informed and Responsive (TIR) Practices

Chapter 3
- Developing Inner Resources
- The Five-Pound Weight Guideline
- The Self-Regulation Scale
- Ground, Breathe, and Orient
- Breathe-With
- De-escalation Protocol—Recognize, Stabilize, and Refer
- Connection—Do Your Students Know How to Ask for Help?

Chapter 4
- Assessment—Are You at Risk for Burnout or Compassion Fatigue?
- Honoring Scope of Practice
- Keep Professional Boundaries
- Daily Mindful Self-Care
- Embodying Your Mindful Self-Care—ARTFUL Self-Care
- A Mindful and Collective Care Meditation
- Creating and Maintaining a Manageable Teaching Schedule
- Ongoing Professional Development and Supervision
- Knowing and Remembering Your WHY

Chapter 5
- Orienting for Safety

Chapter 6
- Seeing Body (PVT) States in the Yoga Session

LIST OF TIR PRACTICES

Chapter 10
- Mindful Listening
- Heartful Listening

Chapter 11
- Nonviolent Communication

Chapter 12
- Trigger and Content Warnings
- Privacy and Discretion
- Inclusive Language
- Responding to Microaggressions
- Mindful Use of Sanskrit
- Indigenous Land Acknowledgment

Chapter 13
- Encourage Choice
- Detailed Class Descriptions and Teacher Bios
- Mindful Use of Your Voice
- Using Clarifying Statements Early in the Class
- Offer Explicit, Ongoing, Informed Consent
- Offering the Choice to Stop
- Invite Students into a Yoga Asana or Practice
- Orient Students Toward Interoception
- Offer Options and Encourage Choice
- Carefully Consider Touch and Hands-on Assists

Chapter 14
- Intentionally Being with What Is There
- Being with the Qualities of Sensations
- Breathing—A Powerful Being-with Practice
- Being with—The Eight Limbs, Grounding, and Breathing
- Being with—Riding the Wave of a Sensation Action Urge
- Being with—Hand over Heart
- Being with—Pendulation
- Being with—Noticing, Naming, and Reorienting Thoughts
- Attuned Teaching

Chapter 15

- Mountain Pose (*Tadasana*)
- Knees to Chest Pose (*Apanasana*)
- Legs up the Wall Pose (*Viparita Karani*)
- Child's Pose (*Balasana*)
- Standing Forward Fold (*Uttanasana*)
- Reclining Bound Angle Pose (*Supta Baddha Konasana*)
- Pyramid Pose (*Parsvottanasana*)
- Warrior Pose 1 (*Virabhadrasana 1*)
- Triangle Pose (*Trikonasana*)
- Belly Breathing
- Sandbag Breathing
- Sighing Breath
- Easy Sitting Pose (*Sukhasana*)
- Nasal Breathing
- Stair-Step Breathing (*Viloma 1*)
- Ratio Breathing
- Chanting Om
- Corpse Pose (*Savasana*)
- Meditation

Chapter 16

- Horse Whinny
- Bellows Breath (*Bhastrika Pranayama*)
- Warrior Pose 2 (*Virabhadrasana 2*)
- Reverse Warrior Pose (*Viparita Virabhadrasana*)
- Modified Side Angle Pose (*Parsvakonasana*)
- Chair Pose (*Utkatasana*)
- Downward-Facing Dog Pose (*Adho Mukha Svanasana*)
- Upward-Facing Dog Pose (*Urdhva Mukha Svanasana*)
- Reverse Table Top Pose (*Ardha Purvottanasana*)
- Baby Cobra Pose (*Ardha Bhujangasana*)
- Block Breathing
- Locust Pose (*Salabhasana*)
- Bridge Pose (*Setu Bandhasana*)
- Modified Camel Pose (*Ustrasana*)
- Plank Pose (*Kumbhakasana*)
- Side Plank Pose (*Vasisthasana*)
- Crescent Lunge Pose (*Anjaneyasana*)

LIST OF TIR PRACTICES

- Boat Pose (*Navasana*)
- Breath of Joy
- Bee Breathing (*Bhramari Pranayama*)
- Lion's Breath (*Simhasana*)
- Shaking
- Standing Squat Pose (*Utkata Konasana*)
- Meditation

Chapter 17

- Tree Pose (*Vrksasana*)
- Alternate Nostril Breathing (*Nadi Shodhanam*)
- Spinal Extension Pose
- Warrior Pose 3 (*Virabhadrasana 3*)
- Seated Twist Pose (*Parivrtta Sukhasana*)
- Alternative Seated Twist Pose (*Bharadvaja's Twist*)
- Reclining Spinal Twist Pose (*Supta Matsyendrasana*)
- Cat Pose (*Bidalasana*)
- Cow Pose (*Bitilasana*)
- Seated Pigeon Pose (*Kapotasana*)
- Pigeon Pose on the Mat
- Reclining Pigeon Pose
- Staff Pose (*Dandasana*)
- Hero Pose (*Virasana*)
- Dancer Pose (*Natarajasana*)
- Eagle Pose (*Garudasana*)
- Lateral Spine Movement
- Balancing Half Moon Pose (*Ardha Chandrasana*)
- Ocean-Sounding Breathing (*Ujjayi Pranayama*)
- Meditation

Chapter 18

- Community Agreements
- Yoga as a Spiritual and Secular Practice
- Creating a Trauma-Informed and Responsive Space

Introduction

atha yogânuåâsanam

Yoga Sutra I:1

OM: Here follows Instruction in Union.

Charles Johnston (1912)

This book was born out of our desire to provide a universal resource for yoga teachers and therapists interested in working within the intersection of trauma-informed (TI) and trauma-responsive (TR) methods and the relational space between yoga and the student. The rapid shifts in research and guidance in the field has created confusion and led to conflicting beliefs about what it means to be a trauma-informed and responsive (TIR) yoga teacher. With the proliferation of 200-hour yoga teacher training, misunderstandings have been passed from teacher to student for at least two decades with a sometimes tenuous connection to best practices and research. Responding to the need, we wrote this book to help define terms, integrate philosophy and science, and offer specific guidelines, practices, and points of inquiry for being trauma-informed.

Being a TIR yoga teacher is not the same as *treating* trauma, or doing what is referred to as *trauma-focused* (TF) work. In TF methods, trauma and trauma-related symptoms are the focus of the methodology. Although it is true that there are yoga protocols and practices designed to specifically support trauma treatment, TIR yoga teaching methods are about your ability to interface with, respond to, and teach all of your students effectively, including those who may have been exposed to trauma. *Being trauma-informed and responsive is about being able to negotiate two truths—yoga can be both a trigger for those who have been traumatized and an effective tool for working with trauma.* This book aims to bring clarity to concepts such as trauma, posttraumatic stress disorder, and TI and TR teaching methods, by integrating the science and theory of trauma with the traditions and practices of yoga. This text will help you gain a clearer understanding of what it means to be a TIR yoga teacher along with practical, step-by-step, accessible teaching points to accomplish this objective. At the same time, you will be encouraged and equipped to connect to yourself and perhaps a therapist as you uncover your own experience of trauma.

This text has been written in the spirit of inquiry. As authors of this text, we endeavored to read the existing literature in the field of trauma and yoga, integrate our findings, and provide an easy-to-use guide for you. We acknowledge there is always more to know and learn. Adherence to a rigid view of right and wrong often gets in the way of what is effective and supportive. Knowledge is always evolving. Our effort has been to create a foundation for all of us to continue to live the question "How can my teaching best serve my students, including those who have experienced trauma?" With more than 50 years of combined yoga practice and 30 years of experience teaching/training yoga teachers, we aim to provide insight into many nuances and subtleties. Yoga falls into the category of learning by doing. When combined with an understanding of one's nervous system regulation and yoga's relationship to it, your teaching comes alive with possibility and healing. We will share research, theory, and our experience. When helpful and relevant, we describe our experiences teaching and administering trauma-informed and trauma-responsive methods in studios, shelters, treatment centers, hospitals, and in the community. In those cases, we will use our initials and pronouns (CCC [she/her] and JS [she/her]).

We are excited to accompany you on your journey as a developing yoga teacher. By the end of this book, we hope being trauma-informed and responsive will be part of your teaching practice's DNA. If you are already a yoga teacher seeking to refine your understanding of trauma-informed and responsive teaching and develop your skills further, we enthusiastically welcome you. Whether you are a seasoned teacher or just learning to teach, integrating TI and TR methods is both easier and harder than you think. We'll let that paradox sink in for a moment... Easier because you may innately feel the call of your nervous system to be more intentional and reflective in your practice. Harder because this type of intentionality and reflection can feel countercultural to productivity (including your yoga practice) and being optimized and efficient in all we do. Being a trauma-informed yoga teacher is much more than simply slowing down and finding a pace consistent with regulating your nervous system. It is about attunement with your nervous system and offering the experience for your students within which they too can practice attunement with their nervous systems. There is more, as you will read in the text, including the key principles of choice, agency, and a felt sense of safety which contribute to trauma-informed teaching.

What to Expect

Using TI and TR methods in your yoga teaching includes many things that are simple to achieve and accessible to all. As you read, you might think, "Well, that's just common sense. I already do that." To which we say, "Great. Keep going, learning, and leading." We have found that common sense is not always so common, and trauma-informed methodology is absent from many teacher training programs. We want to change that with this book. We will cover the common-sense things and look at them through the lens of trauma research, best practices in yoga teaching, and yoga tradition. It is almost impossible to tie all of those things together in a neat package with a bow; however, we believe your teaching and your students will be more emotionally regulated as a result of being trauma-informed and responsive. Perhaps more importantly, you will be more even, psychologically and emotionally regulated, and knowledgeable about the classes you teach. You will wonder more. You will become a keen and curious observer of yourself and your students. For ease of learning, you will notice throughout this book that we will refer to specific ways to make your teaching trauma-informed and responsive.

This is a content warning. This book will include examples of trauma, describe situations that may arise in a yoga setting, and regularly refer to many types of trauma. This is necessary in teaching TI and TR methods. Before you continue, make sure you have the support and resources you need to manage the content present in this book. If you do not, you may want to consider waiting until you do.

How to Use This Book

Reading the book in its entirety will give you the best context of TIR yoga teaching (truth: and it will make us feel better for taking the time to write this book). Your way of being on your yoga mat matters to the yoga class you teach. This book will help you navigate some of the more challenging unseen parts to teaching a yoga class. That said, each chapter is named simply and explicitly so you can follow your curiosities. We will highlight *Trauma-Informed and Responsive Principles for Teaching Yoga*.

INTRODUCTION

These principles are based on therapy, research, and yoga methodology. The principles will help you consolidate your learning and review principles as you refine your teaching skills and share the learnings of this text with others. We have also highlighted *Trauma-Informed and Responsive Practices.* These are active practices that will enhance your TIR yoga teaching. To encourage processing of information, you will find *Journal Prompts* with questions for reflection. Finally, each chapter will conclude with *Teacher Training Discussion Questions.* These questions are designed to help you review the chapter content and initiate discussions. They may also be helpful for teacher training faculty in developing competency assessments.

If you are part of the tl;dr (too long; didn't read) crowd, the teaching points will be essential. No judgments here. We aim to make challenging and complex information accessible and practical for all learning styles so you can be the best yoga teacher you can be. The questions will also stimulate discussion in your yoga teacher training.

This book begins with an introduction that gives you an overview of how we approached this work. The book is then divided into four parts. **Part I** provides the **Foundations of Trauma-Informed and Responsive Yoga Teaching.** Chapters 1 and 2 include defining words and terms that we deem critical for understanding TI and TR methodology. Chapter 3 helps you begin to build your TI and TR toolkit with information on assessing activation, taking a pause, and having a de-escalation protocol. Chapter 4 reviews your mindful self-care. We front-loaded self-care so that you have these tools to support you as you work through sometimes difficult content.

Part II Research and Theory: Embodiment, Polyvagal Theory, and Sensations provides you with the research and theory specific to yoga and trauma. Chapter 5 introduces positive embodiment, interoception, and self-regulation as it relates to you and your teaching. In Chapter 6, the polyvagal theory is explained and discussed in the context of direct application to your teaching. Chapters 7, 8, and 9 cover sensations, a critical component of what is both triggering and healing within yoga practice. You will learn the basics of sensations, their role as communicators, and how sensations inform the process of self-regulation.

Part III Trauma-Informed and Responsive Communication focuses on communication. As yoga teachers, especially TIR yoga teachers, our words are one of our most powerful and potentially harmful tools. Chapter 10 covers communication basics—mindful and heartful listening. Chapter 11 reviews the fundamentals of nonviolent communication. Chapter 12 provides you with invaluable information on content warnings and microaggressions. Last, Chapter 13 details TI and TR cueing and assisting.

Part IV Trauma-Informed and Responsive Yoga Teaching Practices is the work. Chapter 14 will help you explore what it means to teach with self-awareness and attunement and digs into the power of being with what is present in the right here and right now. Chapters 15, 16, and 17 detail the practices that can help your students work with what is present in the moment—practices that soothe and calm, activate and stimulate, and balance and integrate respectively. The final chapter will guide you in cultivating trauma-informed spaces for all bodies.

Embodying Your Learning

We have created journal prompts, teacher training questions, and practices for you to both practice and teach. How much you learn and the nature of that learning will depend on your active engagement in the material and practices.

Take time to journal. Researchers and mental health professionals know that it can be helpful to keep a personal journal in which you can process and reflect upon what you are learning and ground any memories that come up. You might record memories you'd like to talk about with your therapist, particular areas of content of practices that are emotionally challenging for you, and practices that help you self-regulate and calm.

> **Journal Prompt.** Throughout the book, there will be journal prompts offered to help you process the content. They will look like this. The questions will be reflective, asking you to connect the content to your own experience. You can write in your own journal or notebook. We encourage you to take time and complete the journaling tasks. They will help you learn and help you answer the reflective questions at the end of each chapter.

Gather your resources. Tab a section in your journal or create a separate journal called "My Resources." This section can include a list of supportive people and their contact information, calming and grounding practices, as well as tips and practices. You will learn as you read this book what helps you feel self-regulated and ready to learn.

Study Yoga Philosophy, Yoga Texts, and Integrate All Eight Limbs of Yoga
Yoga is a beautiful, spiritual, and holistic mind and body practice. It has eight limbs: Yama (restraints), Niyama (observances), Asana (postures), Pranayama (breathing techniques), Pratyahara (sense withdrawal), Dharana (focused concentration), Dhyana (meditative absorption), and Samadhi (bliss or enlightenment). This text is meant to inform the nature of the teaching of yoga and not to overlap with substantive content in your yoga teacher training. It is critical that you do not consider this text to be a comprehensive guide to yoga teaching. Using this text as a supplement, study and practice the eight limbs of yoga.

Honor Yoga's Roots
Integral to being a TIR yoga teacher is understanding the impact of colonialism and appropriation and its impact in South Asia and effects on what is now understood as yoga. Yoga teachers should educate and inform themselves about the history and roots of yoga and proactively inform their students of the origin of the practices including the lineage, style, and methodology being taught (Yoga Alliance, 2020a). Be sure you understand the difference between cultural appreciation and cultural appropriation, why alcohol and drug use are not appropriate in yoga classes, and how to contextualize yoga artifacts within their rich histories and meanings (Yoga Alliance, 2020a).

Beyond your 200-, 300-, or 500-hour training, continue to study yoga texts. Take continuing education to better understand and honor the roots of yoga. We also encourage you to take classes or training with someone of South Asian heritage. For more on yoga's roots and appropriation, please see:

- *Embrace Yoga's Roots: Courageous Ways to Deepen Your Yoga Practice* by Susanna Barkataki (2020)
- "How can we work together to avoid cultural appropriation?" by Arundhati Baitmangalkar (2023)
- "I teach yoga—its appropriation by the white wellness industry is a form of colonization, but we can move on" by Nadia Gilani (2023)
- *Yoga—Anticolonial Philosophy: An Action-Focused Guide to Practice* by Shyam Ranganathan (2023).

Practice, Practice, Practice
Trauma-informed and responsive yoga teaching is a practice. This text offers many trauma-informed and responsive practices. They will be highlighted for you as you read. You will be encouraged throughout this book to not

only teach, but engage in the practices that are offered. The most effective teachers are those who live and embody what they teach.

What This Book Is Not
This Book Is Not a Book on How to Treat Trauma
If one of your students needs treatment for trauma, that is the purview of a trauma therapist (a specifically trained, licensed mental health professional) or a yoga therapist with trauma training. Later in this book, we will expand on what is referred to as *scope of practice*. Knowing the boundaries of your expertise and the potential harm that can be done when you, or any professional, steps outside of their scope of practice is one of the critical aspects of being trauma-informed.

This Is Not the Book (or Course) on How to Become a Yoga Teacher in Seven Easy Steps
Our intention is that the information from this book will come *alongside* your current yoga teacher training to help you to be as effective as you can be as a leader on your yoga mat. Accordingly, we do not provide an in-depth exploration of yoga philosophy and an all-inclusive list of practices (e.g., mantras, mudras, an expansive list of meditations). This book contains information and explanations to rest upon your existing knowledge of yoga teaching, whatever lineage or style you happen to be training in. We spell out scope of practice as a yoga teacher so you can be comfortable and confident in what you offer the world through your teaching. Whether you are new to teaching yoga or a veteran teacher with lots of experience, you may have already guessed that the journey of becoming a yoga teacher is a lifelong process, in that we are never really done with learning. Part of the teaching journey is remaining open and curious to what is present in front of you now. Our hope is that your journey will be a long and pleasant one full of wonder and gratitude. May it be so. We think yoga teaching is a gift and a calling. We are humbled to be part of your journey.

Case Studies
The case studies in this book are designed to portray the ways in which trauma shows up in the teaching and practice of yoga and to show you how the approaches described herein impact on the people we work with as yoga teachers. We are mindful of the privacy of the people we encounter; with

this in mind, we have included composite accounts and changed details to protect identities.

Closing Acknowledgment and Gratitude

We strongly encourage yoga teachers to engage in a regular practice of acknowledgment of and gratitude for the practice of yoga. Below is a sample acknowledgment and gratitude statement. We end our Introduction and begin our book with this sample from author CCC:

> Yoga philosophy and practice is an ancient
> practice developed in South Asia.
>
> As a practitioner, yoga teacher, yoga therapist, and researcher,
> I am grateful for yoga philosophy and practices.
>
> I am also grateful to those who shared these practices and philosophies
> with my teachers, and to my teachers who shared with me.
>
> I acknowledge that my understanding of yoga, its
> tradition, philosophies, and practices is limited.
>
> I am committed, with humility, to my practice
> and understanding of yoga.

TEACHER TRAINING DISCUSSION QUESTIONS

1. Why is learning how to be a TIR yoga teacher important to you?

2. What do you think led to the Yoga Alliance now requiring 200-hour yoga teacher trainings to include a module on the science of trauma and yoga?

PART I

FOUNDATIONS OF TRAUMA-INFORMED AND RESPONSIVE YOGA TEACHING

CHAPTER 1

Trauma-Informed and Responsive Methods Defined

heyaä duïkham anâgatam

Yoga Sutra II:16

This pain is to be warded off, before it has come.

Charles Johnston (1912)

Trauma-informed and responsive (TIR) care initially evolved from the health care system in recognition of the prevalence of trauma and the association of trauma with psychological and physical difficulties and disorders (Butler *et al.*, 2011). Specifically, the landmark *Adverse Childhood Experiences (ACE) Study* found that early adverse life experiences were associated with adolescent and adult health-risk behaviors and a host of mental and medical health conditions (Felitti *et al.*, 1998). Adverse childhood events (ACEs) are potentially traumatic events that occur during childhood such as experiencing violence, abuse, or neglect, witnessing violence in the home or community, and having a family member attempt or die by suicide (Centers for Disease Control [CDC], 2023a, 2023b). They also include aspects of the child's environments that can undermine the child's feelings of safety and stability such as substance use problems (smoking, heavy drinking, drug use), mental health problems (posttraumatic stress disorder, depression, eating issues), and instability due to parental separation, divorce, or household members being in jail or in prison (CDC, 2023a, 2023b). Over time, the research revealed the following (CDC, 2023a, 2023b):

- ACEs are common: about 61 percent of adults report experiencing at least one ACE before the age of 18.
- Sixteen percent of adults report they have experienced four or

more types of ACEs, with women and several racial/ethnic groups at greater risk for experiencing multiple ACEs.
- Five out of ten of the leading causes of death are associated with ACEs.
- ACEs yield economic and social costs to families, communities, and the larger society in the hundreds of billions of dollars.
- To learn more go to "Take the ACE quiz—and learn what it does and doesn't mean" (Center on the Developing Child, Harvard University; https://developingchild.harvard.edu/media-coverage/take-the-ace-quiz-and-learn-what-it-does-and-doesnt-mean).

The Evolution of Trauma-Informed and Responsive (TIR) Yoga Teaching

Over time, trauma research revealed that, beyond ACEs, trauma was pervasive. In fact, the National Council for Mental Wellbeing reports that 70 percent of adults have experienced some type of traumatic event at least once in their lives (Benjet *et al.*, 2016). The implications for care providers, educators, and yoga teachers are clear—in order to care for and teach individuals effectively, we need to be trauma-informed (Harris & Fallot, 2001). According to Harris and Fallot (2001), to be trauma-informed (TI) is: (1) to understand how violence and victimization have an impact on the lives (and nervous systems) of those with whom we work; (2) to apply that understanding to how we teach and cultivate community to meet the needs and vulnerabilities of those who have been through trauma (Cook-Cottone, 2023; Harris & Fallot, 2001; Spence, 2021). Harris and Fallot (2001) identified five guiding principles: safety, trustworthiness, choice, collaboration, and empowerment. As the field has matured, the principles were updated to include transparency, peer support, mutuality, and voice, and to address cultural, historical, and gender issues (Substance Abuse and Mental Health Services Administration [SAMHSA], 2014). Critically, due to variability and inconsistency in how TI principles were understood and carried out, being trauma-informed did not translate into improved client outcomes (Mersky *et al.*, 2021). From this lack of efficacy, trauma-responsive practices evolved (Mersky *et al.*, 2021). Trauma-responsive (TR) practices are methods nonclinical providers (such as yoga teachers) can use to teach (e.g., trauma psychoeducation), respond to, support, and effectively refer individuals exposed to and affected by trauma.

During these same decades, the interest in yoga was also growing exponentially. Researchers have found that yoga works to reduce the impact of stress by moderating our psychological and physiological stress response systems (Riley & Park, 2015). And we are stressed! Research suggests that the primary reasons people adopt practice include stress relief, relaxation, exercise, depression and anxiety relief, pain relief, physical health issues, and spirituality (Park *et al.*, 2016). According to worldwide yoga statistics (McCain, 2023), more than 300 million people worldwide practice yoga. Between 2010 and 2021, yoga grew in popularity by 63.8 percent with more than 7000 yoga studios in the United States alone, and over 100,000 yoga teachers registered with Yoga Alliance.

This brings us to what we know today. We now know much more about our stress response systems, how trauma affects the body, and how yoga works. *This information can be applied universally through TIR yoga teaching methods.* That means that as we learn and study different lineages of yoga, we can all implement universal, trauma-informed knowledge. We now know what is needed to make sure that those coming to yoga can do so feeling supported and responded to and without being stressed, traumatized, or re-traumatized.

Navigating Terminology: What is Trauma-Informed and Responsive Yoga Teaching?

Let's start with yoga and work our way to TIR methods. Yoga philosophy and practice is an ancient tradition developed in South Asia. As explained in the yoga sutras, yoga is the pathway to actualization of the true self. It is an eight-limb set of practices and philosophies that help you develop a positively embodied life filled with intention, and meaning, or dharma. Through this work, you become more aware of, connected to, and live from an increasingly more integrated sense of who you are and how you are connected to others, all beings, and this world. Yoga practices and teachings were born and continue to evolve within their historical and cultural contexts while shared through texts, mentors, teachers, and schools. Studied and practiced in social and relational contexts, ultimately, yoga is a deeply personal, intimate practice through which we can develop our own relationship with each of the eight limbs in a way that meets us exactly where we are.

> **TIR PRINCIPLE:** YOGA IS PERSONAL
> Yoga is an intimate practice, through which you develop your own relationship with each of the eight limbs in a way that meets you exactly where you are.

TIR methodologies become critical when the yoga teacher, mentor, and/or school enters this relational space, between yoga and the student. This is why being a yoga teacher carries extraordinary responsibility, and our skills, or lack thereof, can have substantial consequences. *It is not yoga, it is us, the teachers of yoga, whose methods for teaching should be trauma-informed and responsive.*

Over the past 20 years, two general definitions of trauma-informed yoga teaching have evolved: trauma-sensitive yoga and TIR yoga teaching. Both approaches emphasize key aspects of yoga delivery such as mindful awareness of body sensations, teaching tools for distress tolerance (e.g., coping), and emphasizing choice and relationship (Cook-Cottone, 2015; Cook-Cottone et al., 2017; Emerson, 2015). There are key distinctions between each approach, including the populations served and methodological nuances such as cueing.

Trauma-sensitive yoga. Trauma-sensitive yoga refers to yoga taught specifically and intentionally to individuals who have been through trauma, with diagnoses of trauma-associated symptoms or posttraumatic stress disorder (PTSD) (Emerson, 2015). Emerson's (2015) text titled *Trauma-Sensitive Yoga in Therapy: Bringing the Body into Treatment* clearly delineates that trauma-sensitive yoga is an adjunct for treatment. Those teaching trauma-sensitive yoga partner with a treatment team treating one's trauma-related symptoms, including medical doctors and mental health professionals. Yoga is seen as a complementary component of treatment. Research done on trauma-sensitive yoga involves participants diagnosed with PTSD. Trauma Center Trauma-Sensitive Yoga (TCTSY) is described as a *specific intervention* for complex trauma or chronic, treatment-resistant PTSD (Emerson, 2015). The TCTSY methods are based on the Hatha style of yoga modified to maximize experiences of self-empowerment while helping students cultivate a positive relationship with their bodies. Emphasis is placed on internal experiences and relationship to one's body. There are no hands-on adjustments or assists. Self-direction and agency are supported as facilitators orient students toward their inner experiences. In addition, facilitators encourage students to use what they notice to inform the choices as they move in their bodies and breathe. Information on training in TCTSY is available at their webpage (www.traumasensitiveyoga.com).

Trauma-informed and responsive yoga teaching. TIR yoga teaching acknowledges that all yoga settings are likely to hold students who have experienced trauma and/or have trauma-related symptomatology. TIR yoga teaching is an approach to teaching yoga in which teachers are trained to have knowledge of trauma and PTSD, the key points of delivering yoga classes relevant to trauma, and scope of practice issues related to the treatment of trauma and provision of yoga (Cook-Cottone *et al.*, 2017). These teachers have learned how to provide a supportive class for individuals experiencing stress or who may have been traumatized (Cook-Cottone *et al.*, 2017). Cues orient students toward self-awareness and interoceptive awareness, emphasize choice and agency, and prioritize safety. TIR teachers are prepared to manage students who may experience trauma symptoms in class. They are knowledgeable and prepared to effectively refer students in need of treatment. TIR yoga teachers are in active engagement in mindful self-care and work on their way of being as an essential aspect of offering trauma-informed yoga sessions (see Figure 1.1).

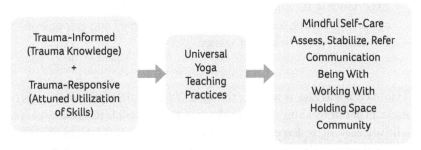

FIGURE 1.1 TRAUMA-INFORMED AND RESPONSIVE YOGA TEACHING PRACTICES

Trauma-informed and responsive yoga teaching is not treatment for trauma. That said, it can be helpful for someone who has been through trauma to go to a yoga class with a TIR yoga teacher. This is because yoga is, at its essence, self-regulating (see sutra 1.2). TIR yoga teaching is *not* a checklist of the things you need to do and say to create absolute safety. Creating absolute safety for all students is impossible. What might feel safe, fun, or comforting for one person may be triggering or upsetting for another. To illustrate, I (CCC) participated in a training related to teaching yoga to individuals who had experienced trauma. There was a strong emphasis on exact words and specific phrases teachers must use. This got the group into a few discussions I could only describe as unresolvable quagmires. For example, the trainees engaged in a debate about verbal cueing. One trainee said, "You should count down for every pose, so students have a sense when the pose will end. This is trauma-informed." Another student responded, "You can't do that! There are veterans who disabled bombs and they counted down, ten, nine, eight [she counted down]…until the bomb either exploded or did not." The conversations spiraled from there.

The truth is, there is no one right thing you can say or do to make a person feel safe. In fact, if you break down the sentence, it is all about you *doing* and *making something happen*. Consider that what is supportive to a student's growth is their own sense of self-determination or agency. Any intervention or support that takes away a student's self-agency won't help. Do countdowns help? I think so—for some. Are they triggering? I think so—for some. There is a Rumi quote that comes to mind: "Somewhere between right and wrong is a garden, I will meet you there." This process is about getting to know your students and working with them in ways that support them. In this way, there is no right or wrong, there is simply what works.

> **TIR PRINCIPLE: CHOICE AND AGENCY**
> Experiencing trauma usually involves lack of choice or personal agency; therefore, teaching in a trauma-informed and responsive way begins with choice and agency.

Trauma is not as rare as we once thought. We can learn a few simple ways to make all of our teaching trauma-informed and accessible to as many people who are seeking it. Experiencing trauma often involves lack of choice or personal agency, therefore teaching in a trauma-informed way begins with choice and agency. That means using invitational language and knowing there are options in how one breathes and does a particular yoga pose. Your instruction needs to be relevant to the bodies in front of you, not how a pose feels in your body or to those in the last class you taught. It can feel very daunting at first to realize that not all bodies can do, as an example, Triangle Pose in the way you were taught (and perhaps love) Triangle Pose.

Like other universal health practices (e.g., washing our hands and brushing our teeth), a universal approach to trauma-informed care is an idea whose time has come. It will allow students to feel supported enough to explore their own body and interior life through yoga practice. We will not inadvertently turn people away who would greatly benefit from the practice. Our teaching is not rigid, unwelcoming, exclusive, unpredictably overstimulating, and/or seemingly full of landmines to a person who is disconnected from their body and perhaps traumatized.

After working through this book, you will be equipped with a toolbox. Consider that some of the people in front of you have struggled with life in some way that has caused deep suffering that they may not even be able to articulate; at times, their suffering may exceed their internal capacity to cope. Trauma is now prevalent enough that the odds of having a traumatized person in any yoga class are high (Cook-Cottone *et al.*, 2017). For this reason alone, we believe it is highly advisable to include some best practices in TIR methods for teaching yoga in all yoga teacher training—even (or especially) at the 200-hour level.

Considering Safety for Your Students and You

We want this experience to feel manageable for you, just as you want your yoga classes to feel accessible and manageable for your students. We are writing this book with you and your students in mind. No matter how strongly we hope you feel safe, how many content warnings we use (more on this later), or how cautious we are, we cannot create a safe experience for *every body*. This is simply a fact.

> **TIR PRINCIPLE: SAFETY**
> Feeling safe is a personal, subjective experience that varies from student to student, minute to minute, pose to pose, and context to context.

In fact, no author, teacher, or trainer can make an experience safe for everyone. Feeling safe is a personal, subjective experience that varies from context to context, pose to pose, minute to minute, and student to student. Each of our bodies has its own unique history of stressors, injuries, and traumas associated with each shape or form our bodies take. A person's sense of safety can shift from one minute to the next depending on a variety of factors such as temperature, the number of people in a room, the presence of a feeling or memory, the words used in a sentence, the sounds from outside the studio, the layout of the doors in and out of a yoga studio, the placement of the yoga mats, lighting, music, and other sounds and/or scents. This is true for the bodies of your yoga students and you.

Just like your yoga students, you need to prioritize your self-care as you make your way through this book. The topics in the book can be stressful and triggering to read, think about, and talk about. You will need a few things to help support your learning process.

Social and mental health support. If you have a history of trauma yourself, consider working with a therapist, trusted friend, or support group while you engage in this content. You will want to have someone to talk to and sufficient social support during times you may feel triggered or old memories come up. If you are unable to find support in your area, consider one of the online counseling platforms such as BetterHelp, PRIDE Counseling, Calmerry, talkspace, Therapy.com, or Free Black Therapy (a nonprofit organization providing therapy for Black and African American individuals). Last, it might be helpful to jot down your local crisis services number, in case you or one of your students is in need. Put all of your resources in the "My Resources" section of your journal (see Introduction).

To be an effective source for referral while granting you an overview of services you may want to explore yourself, it can help to have an understanding of the types of therapy used to treat trauma. Below is a short description of several types of therapy known to be effective (in alphabetical order).

Dialectical Behavior Therapy (DBT) for PTSD is an adaptation of DBT designed for working with individuals who have experienced trauma or have trauma-related symptoms (Bohus et al., 2013; Cook-Cottone, 2023). This multifaceted treatment includes learning and practicing mindfulness skills, tools for emotional regulation and distress tolerance, and strategies for having effective interpersonal relationships (Bohus et al., 2013). DBT for PTSD includes psychoeducation on trauma (learning about trauma, symptoms, and recovery). Uniquely, DBT for PTSD helps patients learn to regulate trauma-associated emotions such as fear, disgust, and powerlessness, while learning how to question non-justified secondary emotions such as guilt, shame, and self-contempt. In addition, DBT for PTSD includes sessions on radical acceptance of trauma-related facts with an inclusion of exposure-based techniques for treatment (Bohus et al., 2013; Cook-Cottone, 2023).

Emotional Freedom Technique (EFT) is an exposure-focused therapy that combines somatic (body/physiological) and cognitive (thinking) elements to manage trauma-related emotions, troubling thoughts, and stress and anxiety. The cognitive elements include self-assessment of one's degree of distress associated with particular memories (0–10). This process includes rehearsing a set-up statement that combines a short description of what is distressing with a self-acceptance statement (e.g., "Even though I have [stated problem], I fully and completely accept myself"). The somatic element involves tapping, with one or two fingers, on various points on the body. Rounds of tapping are completed by repeating the set-up statement three times while tapping on a specific area of the hand and then each of the other points 5–10 times. Each round is followed by a self-assessment until one's distress number is near 0. For more information, see Church (2019).

Eye Movement Desensitization Reprocessing (EMDR) therapy is a structured process that addresses trauma memories focusing on trauma-related body sensation, emotions, and negative self-beliefs (e.g., "I am not safe," "I am not worthy") accompanying periods of bilateral stimulation (BLS; Cook-Cottone, 2023). In BLS, the patient watches a light or object move from side to side, or holds clickers that pulse alternately side to side to produce stimulation on both sides of the body. Deep breathing and self-assessments of distress levels are integrated into the processing sessions. To prepare for this work, preparatory sessions include identifying and installing imagined resources like a safe place, allies, and containers for the feelings which arise from trauma. This installation is completed using BLS. Trauma processing is followed by installing alternative positive beliefs (e.g., "I am worthy of love") using BLS. The EMDR International Association's webpage is www.emdria.org.

Internal Family Systems (IFS) is a form of psychotherapy that helps individuals heal from trauma by accessing and loving their wounded and protected inner parts (Cook-Cottone, 2023). IFS practitioners believe the mind is made of subsystems, or subpersonalities, that interact like members of a family. These family members include the core self, managers, firefighters, and exiles (Cook-Cottone, 2023). The main focus of IFS is to heal one's wounded parts and restore mental balance by working with the dynamics between the parts while developing a person's core sense of self. See more at https://ifs-institute.com.

Trauma-Focused Cognitive Behavioral Therapy (TF-CBT) involves working with one's thoughts, feelings, and behaviors. With a therapist, individuals explore how thoughts, feelings, and behaviors may have been affected by traumatic experience(s) and symptoms. Generally, CBT approaches include psychoeducation about trauma (learning about trauma and its effects) and identifying the negative beliefs that may be associated with trauma. For example, common trauma-related thoughts include "I am helpless or powerless" and "I am not worthy." This type of therapy also helps individuals address managing emotions, learning about how emotions and thoughts deeply affect each other with the integration of coping and relaxation strategies (Cook-Cottone, 2023). TF-CBT can occur in two ways. First, Exposure Therapy (ET) involves a gradual desensitization to trauma memories and triggers by talking about them, imagining them, and sometimes recreating aspects of them (the sounds or images). Note, there are many practitioners who do not believe this type of treatment is necessary or appropriate for all patients. Second, Cognitive Processing Therapy (CPT) works with trauma memories with a specific focus on how the memory has affected beliefs about the self, others, and the world. For example, trauma-related beliefs about the self may present as "I am not safe," about others as "You can't trust anyone," and about the world as "The world is a dangerous place." CPT also helps individuals explore how trauma-related beliefs shape emotions and behaviors (Cook-Cottone, 2023). Finally, this approach to treatment involves the development of more positive beliefs (e.g., "I can learn how to create safety in my life," "There are people you can trust," and "I can learn how to be effective and safe in this world") which supports the selection of effective and healthy coping behaviors. The TF-CBT webpage has a "Find a Therapist" section (see https://tfcbt.org).

Written Exposure Therapy (WET) is a five-session exposure-based intervention based on the work of Dr. James Pennebaker (Thompson-Hollands et al., 2019). Sessions include psychoeducation on PTSD and how writing about trauma helps in recovery. There are 30-minute periods during which patients are told to write about specific details, emotions, and sensory experiences associated with the event. Writing sessions are followed by a check-in with the therapist surrounding the patient's reactions to writing about the experience. For more about WET for PTSD, read Sloan and Marx (2019).

Yoga Therapy. According to the International Association of Yoga Therapists (IAYT), Yoga Therapy is a process through which a yoga therapist provides typically one-on-one instruction in yogic practices and teachings to prevent or alleviate pain and suffering and their root causes. Yoga Therapy has been used to support those who are suffering with trauma-related symptoms in their recovery. To find a yoga therapist, go to the IAYT webpage and search the Certified Yoga Therapist database (www.iayt.org).

TIR methods for teaching yoga can support both the teacher and student(s) during a yoga session. There is a growing body of practice, theory, and research that supports these methods as foundational. Trauma-informed methods are about creating an accepting, compassionate, and inclusive environment for students to practice yoga; distinct from treatment and methods used in yoga taught as an adjunct to or complementary therapy in treatment. You, as the yoga teacher, will play a crucial role in helping your student(s) learn self-regulating practices that feel manageable and safe in their bodies. You will also be ready to facilitate referral for those students who need support.

TEACHER TRAINING DISCUSSION QUESTIONS

1. What are the ACEs and why are they important to trauma-informed yoga teachers?
2. Coming from a place of inquiry and curiosity, how may your understanding of what it means to be a trauma-informed and responsive (TIR) teacher be shifting?
3. What does the term "Universal" practice mean to you?
4. What is the difference between trauma-sensitive yoga and TIR methods for teaching yoga? Acknowledge the population, function, and methods.
5. Can a yoga teacher create a completely safe environment for everyone? Why or why not?

CHAPTER 2

Trauma Basics and Terminology

dëg-daråana-åaktyor ekâtmatevâsmitâ

Yoga Sutra II:6

Self-assertion [false identity] comes from thinking of the Seer [self as witness] and the instrument of vision as forming one self.

Charles Johnston (1912)

Foundational to being a trauma-informed and responsive (TIR) yoga teacher is understanding what trauma is, the effects of trauma, the symptoms and presentation of posttraumatic stress disorder (PTSD), and what trauma might look like within the context of a yoga class or session. As in the yoga sutra above, Desikachar (1995) reminds us not to make assumptions as mood, habits, and surroundings are ever changing and connected to the eternal source. This chapter reveals the impact trauma can have on a person's physiology, emotions, thoughts, and behaviors. It allows us to understand other people's attempts at coping, management, and getting by without judgment. More, it sets the stage for how we can respond to these attempts by offering acceptance and support. In this chapter, we will review trauma basics and terminology used in yoga settings to describe trauma-informed methods. This includes defining trauma and reviewing the causes and maintaining factors in trauma symptoms. We will also review terminology such as trauma-sensitive yoga and trauma-informed methods for teaching yoga.

What Is Trauma?

Life is a process of meeting our own needs, wants, and dharma (our life's work), while navigating the supports and challenges the world presents.

Trauma occurs when the world's presented challenges are greater than what your system can effectively manage (Cook-Cottone, 2023). Potentially traumatizing events (PTEs) can include direct exposure to death, serious injury, sexual violence, the threat of death, serious injury, and/or sexual violence (American Psychiatric Association, 2022). These events can also include witnessing a traumatic event, learning that a relative or close friend was exposed to trauma, and/or indirect exposure to traumatic details of an event (American Psychiatric Association, 2022).

We call them potentially traumatizing events because no one event or type of event will affect all individuals in the same way. Trauma is not defined by the event; rather, it is defined by the event's *impact* on our nervous systems. Our bodies, inclusive of our nervous systems, do the very best they can to keep us safe and functioning (Cook-Cottone, 2023). We were all born with a stress management and trauma response system. The good news is that, most of the time, these systems work very well, assisting us to manage stress and effectively cope with potentially traumatizing events.

> **TIR PRINCIPLE:** TRAUMA AND IMPACT
> Trauma is not defined by the event; it is defined by the impact of the event on the nervous system.

When the *experience* of stress and trauma overwhelms the nervous system's ability to cope, the person exposed may experience feelings of helplessness, powerlessness, incapacitation, and terror. During the potentially traumatizing event, the body can go into shock brought on by a sudden drop in blood flow through the body. Symptoms include dizziness, light-headedness, anxiety, confusion, excessive sweating, shallow breathing, shaking, pale and clammy skin, and blueing/graying lips and fingernails. Shock is a serious condition, can exacerbate the effects of the event, and requires medical support. Whether or not shock occurs, trauma and stress can cause the nervous system to move into a prolonged stress response, prioritizing safety and protection over all else (Cook-Cottone, 2023). Symptoms can range from increased sensitivity and reactivity to clinical mental health disorders. When and how this happens is different for everyone, and countless factors play a role. Some factors relate specifically to your individual and internal experiences, interacting in ways that may promote risk or enhance resilience (see Figure 2.1).

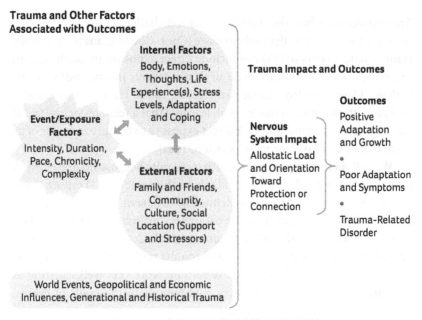

FIGURE 2.1 CAUSES AND EFFECTS OF TRAUMA

Internal Factors

Internal, or individual, factors include physiological components such as the overall sensitivity and resilience of the nervous system, wellbeing and health, level of nourishment, and level of or access to rest and restoration. Illness, both acute and chronic, can add risk. In some cases, medical experiences can result in risk for trauma (surgery, invasive treatments). Emotional factors can also contribute, including mental health status (e.g., depression, anxiety, or other mental health concerns) and emotion regulation skills. Cognitive functioning, or how someone thinks through stress and life events, can also make a difference. Personal life experience leading up to the trauma can play a role. For example, experiences such as being placed in foster care can promote risk, while being raised in a loving and supportive home can promote resilience. Affecting all of these layers of self is the personal, lifelong exposure to stress and trauma as it affects the nervous system and is held in the body as chronic or habitual patterns of bodily reaction or protection. Personal resilience and risk are related to a person's coping resources and skills as well as their system's ability to adapt to stress and potentially traumatizing experiences.

Last, many experience *intergenerational trauma*, or the effects of trauma experienced by your parents and possibly their parents, leaving your nervous system sensitive and/or heightened to potential threats (Yehuda &

Lehrner, 2018). Resemaa Menakem (2017) refers to this type of trauma as a *soul wound*—a wound that travels through families as one family member abuses another, through unsafe and abusive systems and cultural norms, and through the genetic expression of trauma from one generation to the next (p. 10).

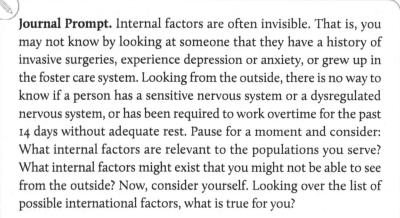

Journal Prompt. Internal factors are often invisible. That is, you may not know by looking at someone that they have a history of invasive surgeries, experience depression or anxiety, or grew up in the foster care system. Looking from the outside, there is no way to know if a person has a sensitive nervous system or a dysregulated nervous system, or has been required to work overtime for the past 14 days without adequate rest. Pause for a moment and consider: What internal factors are relevant to the populations you serve? What internal factors might exist that you might not be able to see from the outside? Now, consider yourself. Looking over the list of possible international factors, what is true for you?

External Factors

External factors also play a role. External factors can include the level of support or stress experienced within one's family or household. Some families have warm and supportive households, whereas other households can feel like dangerous, unpredictable places. For example, in some homes, family members are beaten, abused, and neglected, while in other homes, family members are reliably loved, personal boundaries are respected, and each person experiences a sense of personal agency and self-determination. Other factors like access to water, plumbing, heat and shade, and the safe means for preparing food contribute to risk and resilience.

Types of trauma common in this domain include domestic violence, neglect, physical abuse, and sexual abuse. When abuse is chronic, invasive, and interpersonal in nature, it is referred to as *complex trauma*. Complex trauma consists of exposure to multiple traumatic events that are of a personal and interpersonal nature (see the National Child Traumatic Stress Network at www.nctsn.org). If complex trauma occurs in childhood, it can be particularly difficult to manage because quite often caregivers who were meant to keep a child safe were either the perpetrator of the trauma or complicit in it. Developmental trauma is also within this domain. It occurs when there is repeated trauma and loss within a child's primary relationships early in development. Both complex and developmental trauma can affect the development of trust, a personal sense of safety, and formation of a sense of self—an identity with a sense of personal boundaries and self-determination.

Community factors play a role. Some communities have easy access to food, safe places to gather and interact, mental health supports and therapy, yoga and other mind-body practices, schools with adequate funding and engaged and supported teachers, as well as grocery stores, libraries, parks, and gardens. Many do not. Natural disasters (earthquakes, hurricanes, drought, fire) can impact a community and cause trauma. Work community and daily tasks can also contribute to risk. Soldiers know this all too well. This can also be true for individuals who work with others who have been exposed to trauma. Hearing of the trauma of others, over and over, can begin to impact the nervous system much like direct exposures; this is called *vicarious trauma*.

The larger culture can perpetuate trauma, including one's access to human rights and fundamental resources. Systemic trauma occurs when institutions and/or the leadership within institutions engage in practices that cause harm (physiological, emotional, spiritual, physical, or sexual) to specific individuals or groups.

> Trauma is a constitutive element of intersectional oppression experienced by individuals whose developmental and life trajectories have been sabotaged by health disparities, human right violations, bigotry, colonial structures of power, social inequalities and extreme poverty amongst others. (Liasidou, 2022, p. 3)

For example, for some students, systemically underfunded educational systems and instructional practices can create risk for trauma. Prison systems are also known for their potentially traumatizing conditions. It is well known that those with developmental disabilities and those within the geriatric age group are at risk. At the community level, events that occur within (or to) communities such as racially motivated and targeted shootings can leave entire neighborhoods and cities in fear and conflict for years. For communities that have been marginalized by the dominant culture, risk increases with chronic exposure to oppressive beliefs such as ableism, classism, ageism, homophobia, misogyny, racism, sexism, transphobia, heterosexism, xenophobia, and beliefs and biases related to religion. Identity trauma refers to the increased frequency and severity of trauma based on identity, especially subordinated and marginalized identities.

TRAUMA BASICS AND TERMINOLOGY

External factors can also exist in a more global and pervasive manner affecting all people or differentially affecting specific groups of people (e.g., certain geographic or impoverished areas). These include global world events, geopolitical influences, as well as the generational and historical effects trauma can have on descendants. Examples include war, famine, international sanctions, terrorism, mass shootings, gender-based violence, and human trafficking. Systemically embedded discriminatory systems manifesting in laws and government policy facilitate higher risk for specific citizens to experience trauma (e.g., gender-based laws, laws discriminating against specific ethnic/racial groups). This is a source point for generational embodiment of historical trauma.

Journal Prompt. What external factors may affect the yoga students you hope to or do work with? What have you noticed among your students that may suggest the effects of this type of trauma? When you look at your own history and context, are there external factors that have affected your wellbeing? In what ways?

TIR PRINCIPLE: TRAUMATIC EXPOSURE VARIES
Traumatic exposure varies by intensity, duration, frequency, pace, chronicity, breadth, and complexity.

Event/Exposure Factors
Intensity, duration, frequency, pace, chronicity, breadth, and complexity of exposure to stress and trauma also have an impact. All of these factors contribute to risk or resilience.

Table 2.1 Event and Exposure Factors Contributing to Risk of Trauma Symptomatology

Event/Exposure Factors	Description and Examples
Intensity	Refers to the strength or magnitude of a traumatic event and can range from low intensity (a family member is hospitalized for a curable condition) to high intensity (sexual abuse or a fatal accident).

cont.

TRAUMA-INFORMED AND TRAUMA-RESPONSIVE YOGA TEACHING

Event/Exposure Factors	Description and Examples
Duration	Refers to the length of the exposure. For example, a violent storm might last a matter of hours with no reprieve, while a robbery on the street or car accident might last less than 120 seconds.
Frequency	Refers to how many times potentially traumatizing events occur over a period of time. Some experience potentially traumatizing events only once, while others may face multiple events in their lifetimes. For example, sexual abuse can be a one-time event or occur over a period of years.
Pace	Refers to how often a person is exposed to a potentially traumatizing event. For example, an individual might be exposed to three or four stressful events over a period of ten years, whereas another might be forced to navigate the nightly drunken rages of an abusive parent or partner.
Chronicity	Refers to how long a person is exposed to potentially traumatizing experience over time. This can vary from a short exposure (a car accident) to long-term exposure (chronic domestic violence, a decade of war).
Breadth	Refers to the degree to which the potentially traumatizing event is localized or broad. For example, a single car accident in which an individual's partner is killed is more localized. In contrast, a lethal earthquake caused driving bans and electric outages, while grounding 911 workers and eliminating access to hospitals for tens of thousands of people for several days.
Complexity	Refers to multiple traumatic events that are invasive and interpersonal. For example, war, familial sexual or physical abuse, domestic violence, torture, sex trafficking, or slavery.

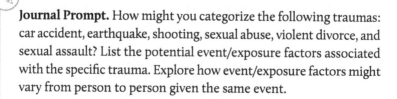

Journal Prompt. How might you categorize the following traumas: car accident, earthquake, shooting, sexual abuse, violent divorce, and sexual assault? List the potential event/exposure factors associated with the specific trauma. Explore how event/exposure factors might vary from person to person given the same event.

The Effects of Trauma

Years of research on adversity and trauma have revealed that exposure is not rare, and the effects are both mental and physical, varying substantially from person to person. Exposure to potentially traumatizing events is dysregulating to the nervous system (Cook-Cottone, 2023). As highlighted above, the various factors (internal, external, and event/exposure factors) contribute to outcomes. Individuals chronically exposed to stress and trauma are at higher risk for stress-related illness and mental health difficulties.

Nervous system impact and outcomes. There are two ways one's nervous system is impacted by stressors and trauma—allostatic load and an orientation shift toward protection. The shifts in allostatic load are important to consider; they can create a foundation of resilience or, over time, be the cause of vulnerability and risk for poor outcomes.

Stress and allostatic load. Guidi and colleagues (2020) describe allostatic load as the burden of chronic stress and life events, and its impact on the body's physiological systems. To break it down: stress happens, and the body responds by taking on the allostatic load. This means the body is gearing up to handle the stress. It does this by activating the cardiovascular, neuroendocrine, and central nervous systems while deactivating the immune system. Immune system suppression allows the body to allocate all of its energy to responding effectively to the stressors. Given adequate support and time to recover and cope, the body is able to return to typical functioning. The cardiovascular, neuroendocrine, and central nervous systems all return to normal, and the immune system begins to function as usual.

An important caveat: your own behaviors can cause you stress. For example, your body and brain experience drinking alcohol as a stressor to manage. The same is true for other behaviors that people often engage in as attempts to deal with life stress (e.g., smoking, over-exercising, and over-working). Consider these two scenarios:

> Scenario 1: You have a really hard day at work and feel completely depleted, so you come home and have a few glasses of wine to relax. Your body now has two stressors to manage: your work-related stress and the stress of managing the alcohol you ingested. You wake up still feeling depressed, dehydrated, and potentially hungover.
>
> Scenario 2: You have a really hard day at work and feel completely depleted. You register for yoga in the morning, eat a nutritious meal, take a bath or shower, and then settle in with a cup of herbal tea to read, watch a show, or journal. You wake up concerned about work, though a bit restored. You grab your yoga mat and head off to class.

Without sufficient time to rest and restore, the allostatic load response can become *allostatic overload* when the body can no longer handle the stress, cope, or adapt. Allostatic overload can perpetuate physical disease, mental health issues, and an inability to successfully manage everyday life. It can leave you at high risk for trauma-related symptoms and disorders (e.g., PTSD, depression, and anxiety).

> **Journal Prompt.** How do you manage stress? Do your go-to ways of handling stress restore you or further deplete you? What role does your yoga practice play in your stress management? What role might your yoga classes play in your students' attempts to manage the stress in their lives?

Connection and protection. Our nervous systems are hard-wired to keep us safe, to protect us. For most of us, this is well balanced with a drive to connect, learn, and experience all of the beautiful things life has to offer. With exposure to adversity and potentially traumatizing events, however, our nervous systems become increasingly oriented toward safety and protection. In some cases, we may begin perceiving almost everything as a threat (Cook-Cottone, 2023). Ultimately, outcomes include poor adaptation, trauma-related symptoms, and trauma-related disorders (see Figure 2.1 Causes and Effects of Trauma). Importantly, there is also a chance for positive adaptation and growth (Wu *et al.*, 2019).

Poor adaptation and symptoms. Back to the Adverse Childhood Events (ACEs) study (Felitti *et al.*, 1998; see Chapter 1). It is theorized that exposure to ACEs is stressful and can facilitate disrupted neurodevelopment. These disruptions show up as difficulty learning, difficulty engaging with the environment, hyperactivity, depression, and anxiety-related disorders. Over time, social, emotional, and cognitive impairment can lead to adoption of health-risk behaviors such as smoking, substance use, and poor sexual decision making. These behaviors increase risk of disease and mortality. Those with ACEs were at increased risk for early death. Alarmingly, those with six or more ACEs were found to have higher odds of dying up to 20 years earlier than those with none.

Trauma-related disorder. Exposure to potentially traumatizing experiences can result in mental disorders, including elevated risk of anxiety and depressive disorders (Gluck *et al.*, 2021; Juruena *et al.*, 2020) as well as trauma and stress-related disorders, such as PTSD. PTSD is a life-disrupting disorder that occurs following exposure to a potentially traumatizing event (American Psychiatric Association, 2022). There are four core symptoms: re-experiencing, avoiding reminders, negative thoughts and feelings, and hyperarousal and reactivity (American Psychiatric Association, 2022). Some people who experience PTSD also have dissociative symptoms. It is crucial that yoga teachers are able to recognize symptoms related to trauma exposure to effectively support and refer potentially traumatized students.

Table 2.2 shows each of the core areas of symptoms including dissociative symptoms. Each section incorporates some of the possible ways specific symptoms might show up in class. Without solid training in trauma-informed yoga teaching, it can be easy to see symptoms of trauma as resistance or indicators of difficult students. Knowing the symptoms and how they might be displayed in class can help you, as a yoga teacher, be more accepting and compassionate.

Table 2.2 Symptoms Related to Trauma Exposure

Type of Symptom	Symptoms and Possible Presentation in Yoga Class
Re-experiencing	• Upsetting and unwanted memories of the event • Nightmares associated with the trauma • Flashbacks (reliving or feeling like it is happening right now) • Emotional and physical distress after exposure to reminders of trauma • Physical reactivity and distress after exposure to reminders of trauma • Reenactment behavior—the unconscious repetition of aspects of your trauma in your day-to-day life **Possible presentation in a yoga class:** distress, tears, suddenly leaving class, staying in Child's Pose to hide tears or anxiety, non-responsiveness to teacher cues, and sudden agitation or behavior that seems out of context.
Avoiding Trauma Reminders	• Avoidance of trauma-related thoughts (trying not to think about it) • Avoidance of trauma-related feelings • Avoidance of trauma-related reminders **Possible presentation in a yoga class:** lack of responsiveness to teacher cues, seemingly resistant, intense engagement in postures or alignment, pushing too hard, difficulty settling in quieter and restorative poses, leaving before *Savasana*, choosing a place in class with minimal stimuli (a corner spot, back row), inconsistent attendance.

cont.

Type of Symptom	Symptoms and Possible Presentation in Yoga Class
Thoughts or Feelings	*Thoughts* • Difficulty remembering key features of the trauma • Negatively skewed thoughts and assumptions about self, others, and the world • Few or limited thoughts about the future • Exaggerate blame of self or others related to the trauma • Decreased interest in activities • Cycling between overwhelming and constrictive thoughts • Increased disbelief, denial, rumination, and obsession *Feelings* • Negative affect such as anger, sadness, contempt, disgust, fear, guilt, shame, hopelessness • Fear of going crazy or "losing it" • Feeling isolated or alone • Difficult feeling positive affect such as happiness, cheerfulness, pride, and joy **Possible presentation in a yoga class:** pessimistic about skills and learning, seemingly resistant, may speak negatively about the studio or other students, over-apologizes for small things (being late, trouble with the webpage), overly compliant, inconsistent attendance, seems lost in thoughts, appears to be angry or upset much of the time, is a loner, and rarely smiles or laughs.
Hyperarousal and Reactivity	*Hyperarousal* • Hypervigilance • Exaggerated startle response • Cycling between body tension/activation and shutdown • Trouble concentrating • Difficulty sleeping *Reactivity* • Severe physical reactions to something that reminds you of the trauma • Irritability and aggression • Self-destructive, destructive, reckless, or risky behavior • Chronic body tensions and activation or shutdown and deactivation **Possible presentation in a yoga class:** finds a location where they can see the door and no one can be behind them, resistant about moving mat, reactive or easily agitated, pushes too hard, does not consistently respond to cues, moves to advanced poses without mastery of more basic poses (throwing self into handstand), seems tense even in restorative poses, does not or is reluctant to close eyes.

TRAUMA BASICS AND TERMINOLOGY

Dissociative Symptoms	• Depersonalization—feeling detached from oneself, like an observer in a dream • No sense of self (Who am I?) • Derealization—feeling a sense of unreality, distance, or distortion as if things are not real **Possible presentation in a yoga class:** doesn't seem to be completely present, may miss or not respond to cues, does not connect with other students or you as a teacher, appears aloof or disinterested, can seem bored or distracted, may not notice the impact of behaviors on others (spraying a scent on mat during class, coming in late and placing mat in the middle of class), has difficulty settling in for *Savasana* or skips it.

Journal Prompt. How might a yoga student demonstrate each of the symptom areas in yoga class? What might you notice as a teacher? If a yoga teacher did not know about the symptoms of trauma, how might these symptoms (e.g., resistance or shutdown) be misinterpreted and misunderstood?

Positive adaptation and growth. Some individuals exposed to trauma positively adapt and experience growth. *Posttraumatic growth* is positive psychological changes sustained after experiencing trauma (Wu *et al.*, 2019). When confronting life-threatening events, individuals who experience posttraumatic growth reassess their goals and priorities, have a greater appreciation of life, and experience a shift in spirituality and relationship enhancement (Tedeschi *et al.*, 2017). After trauma, researchers report that anywhere from 10 percent to 77 percent of those exposed may experience posttraumatic growth, with a little over 50 percent experiencing moderate to high posttraumatic growth (Morrison & Dwarika, 2022; Wu *et al.*, 2019).

> **TIR PRINCIPLE: POSTTRAUMATIC GROWTH**
> Posttraumatic growth is possible, and yoga can help.

Posttraumatic growth is well aligned with yoga concepts and practices (see Table 2.3). Your trauma-informed yoga teaching can support your students' pathway to posttraumatic growth.

Table 2.3 Posttraumatic Growth and Yoga

Area of Posttraumatic Growth	Yoga Concepts and Possible Presentation in Yoga Class
Appreciation of Life	Mindfulness, gratitude, ability to be present and stay present to what is in front of you
Enhanced Relationship with Others	Loving-kindness, yoga community, service, self-awareness, self-care, ability to form secure attachments, increasing tolerance for discomfort, healthy boundary setting
Spiritual Change	Connection to others through a sense of common humanity, establishing a sense of safety in your own body, self-compassion and compassion for others, a sense of interconnectedness with other sentient beings, and a oneness with nature
Development of Personal Strengths	Practice developing inner self-regulation for emotions and distress, minimizing unhelpful responses to memories or triggers, ability to have a one-pointed focus, improved concentration, and practice detaching from the material
New Possibilities in Life	Dharma, gaining a different perspective

How Many People Have Been Exposed to Trauma?

Studies of adult exposure to trauma show wide ranges of rates across countries. For example, in a worldwide study of trauma exposure, the World Mental Health Survey Consortium found that, among the countries reporting, anywhere from 29 percent to 83 percent of the adult population reported exposure to a traumatic event (Benjet *et al.*, 2016). The United States Centers for Disease Control (CDC) reports that more than 1 in 3 women and 1 in 4 men experience sexual violence involving physical contact in their lifetime. In addition, 1 in 4 girls and 1 in 13 boys experience sexual abuse.

Among those exposed to traumatic events, only a percentage are diagnosed with PTSD. Koenen and colleagues (2017) report that the cross-national lifetime prevalence of PTSD is about 3.9 percent. Among individuals exposed to a traumatic event, the rate of PTSD is a little higher at 5.6 percent. These rates cannot be generalized. Rates can be much higher for those who are exposed to systemic inequalities, gender-based violence, terrorism, war, racism, and child sexual abuse, and those with multiple trauma exposures. For example, in a study of 7000 predominantly African American women of low socioeconomic status (SES), over 90 percent of the women reported significant trauma, just over 30 percent met criteria for major depressive disorder, and 32 percent met criteria for PTSD (Gluck *et al.*, 2021).

Interestingly, an evolving body of research suggests yoga and other physical activity may play a role in posttraumatic growth (e.g., Zhang *et al.*, 2022).

> **TIR PRINCIPLE:** TRAUMA IS UNIVERSAL
> Trauma is a universal experience affecting people across cultures, countries, races and ethnicities, incomes, gender identities, and ages.

That said, if you are teaching in a yoga studio, given the rates of trauma exposure and sexual and physical abuse, it is likely that up to 50 percent of students will have a trauma history. If you are teaching in a community setting in an area with known poverty and neighborhood violence, you can expect that a majority of your students will have experienced trauma.

Trauma-informed and responsive means you have studied and know this information about trauma and what it can look like in a student. It also means you know what to do, and how to do it, when trauma symptoms show up in your class. TIR yoga teaching is an implicit practice that involves a balance between your own self-awareness and presence and your mindful awareness of and attunement with your students. Your mindful awareness, presence, and attunement offers students a chance to *co-regulate*. That means that within the context of *your* self-regulated embodiment and teaching, students can ultimately internalize a sense of safety and trust, and begin to befriend their bodies. This is the work you will find in the forthcoming chapters of this book.

TEACHER TRAINING DISCUSSION QUESTIONS

1. What are some of the causes of trauma?
2. Name and define some different types of trauma.
3. Why do we use the term "potentially traumatizing events" (PTEs)?
4. What are the event/exposure variations of trauma? How might their impact vary from person to person given the same or similar event?
5. What are the effects of trauma? What might you notice in your yoga class?

6. What is the likelihood you will be teaching yoga to someone with trauma? Does this change for community classes, prison yoga, yoga in hospitals, yoga in schools, or yoga in domestic violence shelters? What is the likelihood that you will be teaching yoga to someone who has experienced trauma where you teach or would like to teach yoga?

CHAPTER 3

Preparedness—Resource, Assess, Pause, De-escalate, and Connect

tatra sthitau yatno 'bhyâsaï

Yoga Sutra I:13

The right use of the will is the steady effort to stand in spiritual being [practice].

Charles Johnston (1912)

This chapter is early in the book so that you have tools to come to emergency assistance for those who are having difficulty. These include tools for resourcing, assessment, taking a pause, de-escalation, and connection. Despite our focus on our students, trauma-informed and responsive (TIR) teacher training can bring up our own old wounds and traumas. The TIR guiding values here are empowerment, support, and choice (SAMHSA, 2014). This chapter serves the dual purpose of making sure you are prepared if anything comes up in your training, while preparing you to support your students more effectively going forward.

> **TIR PRINCIPLE: DEVELOP INNER RESOURCES**
> Encourage the development of inner resources, or internal aids, that you can turn to when you need support.

TIR PRACTICE: DEVELOPING INNER RESOURCES

Trauma can feel incapacitating and erode trust in yourself. Yoga practice helps you develop inner resources. These are resources that are provided by your own mind and personal capacities, and developed and strengthened through practice (Cook-Cottone, 2023; Taylor, 2021). They are internal aids you can turn to when you need support. Inner resources come in many shapes and sizes. They include mindset, the four immeasurables (compassion, joy, equanimity, and loving-kindness), mindful attitudes (curiosity, openness, acceptance, allowing), and somatic skills (breathwork, orienting, and grounding; Cook-Cottone, 2015, 2023; Taylor, 2021). They can include imagined sanctuaries, such as a safe place you mentally construct (or remember) that you can recall in times of distress. Inner resources can have a spiritual quality to them including your inner connection to the God of your understanding, those who have passed away and now serve as inner guides, or the images of animals that hold the qualities that soothe and support you (e.g., a lion for courage, a wild horse for the feeling of freedom and power). Each time you call on your resources when you sit to meditate, spend time being with a difficult sensation or emotion, breathe through a challenge, upsetting thought, or memory, or press your feet into the ground, engage your core, and reach powerfully, you are building your capacity for resilience and inner strength. You are building your inner resources.

You can help your yoga students develop their inner resources informally through cueing to practices like pressing your feet into the floor for a sense of grounding during a pose or orienting to breath during a challenging pose. You can help develop inner resources through more formal practices such as a yoga workshop or class designed specifically to support the development of inner resources, taking time to define inner resources and guide students to identify and practice using them. The practice of Yoga Nidra is another formalized way to help students develop inner resources (for more on this, see Miller, 2022). As you build your inner resources, you might add notes to your "My Resources" section of your journal or notebook (see Introduction).

> **Journal Prompt.** Take a moment to reflect on your inner resources. Jot down those that come to mind. How often do you turn to them and in what contexts? How might you further their development? Last, how might the development of inner resources support your students?

TIR PRACTICE: THE FIVE-POUND WEIGHT GUIDELINE

The five-pound weight is a sharing technique often helpful when conducting or taking TIR training. Five pounds is a metaphor for a manageable experience you might share. Imagine that you are at the gym and pick up a five-pound weight. You can do many repetitions, curling the weight toward your shoulder using your biceps. Since the weight is manageable, you keep your form and stay steady. Now, if you switched to a 40-pound weight, perhaps there are some of you who could do a few repetitions without losing form; most certainly I (CCC) could not. I would likely struggle with one repetition and then utterly lose my form and integrity trying to lift it to my shoulder a second time.

When you are in TIR training, it is good to share and use examples similar to the five-pound weight. It is enough weight that you can feel it and practice being with it, yet it does not cause overwhelm or loss of control, or create risk. We can learn a lot by working with our five-pound weights in life: the time our friend did not show up to coffee, the failed paper at school, the loss of a championship game, or hurtful words exchanged between friends. These are helpful, low-cost narratives within which we can practice sharing and coping. I (CCC) have found that when students or facilitators begin to share their very personal and traumatic stories—those at a 40-pound weight equivalent or more—it can be quite overwhelming for those in the training. It is often much too big emotionally to feel manageable, while learning and practicing new skills. If during your training you feel 40-, 50-, 250-, and 1000-pound memories are coming up and fostering feelings of dysregulation, this might be a good time to seek a therapist or get additional help from your loved ones. If these continuously emerge in your training, it is time to take a pause and address the issue. TIR yoga teacher training should not be confused with therapeutic interventions in which traumas are shared and processed.

Assess: How Regulated Are You and Your Students?

TIR yoga teaching requires the ability to be mindfully aware of levels of nervous system activation and regulation of both yourself and your students. Over the span of a day (sometimes even an hour), your activation level can vary from very calm and relaxed to extremely activated and reactive. Mindful awareness of your level of activation and regulation is powerful. Awareness is essential for attunement with, and care of, self and others. Mindful awareness enables you to effectively respond to what is needed rather than reacting to the state of your nervous system.

TRAUMA-INFORMED AND TRAUMA-RESPONSIVE YOGA TEACHING

> **TIR PRINCIPLE: SELF-REGULATION SCALE**
> Use the self-regulation scale to assess your state and the state of your students.

TIR PRACTICE: THE SELF-REGULATION SCALE

Throughout this book, we will refer to the self-regulation scale (see Figure 3.1). On one end, lower numbers refer to a relaxed and calm state of being. On the other end, higher numbers reflect a state of activation and overwhelm. You will want to notice both the regulation level (e.g., "I am at about a 5 or 6") along with your directionality (e.g., "I am on my way to a 7 or 8" or "I was a 7 and I'm now at 5 or 6; I can feel myself calming down"). It is helpful to intentionally pause through your yoga sessions or classes to assess where you and your students are on the scale.

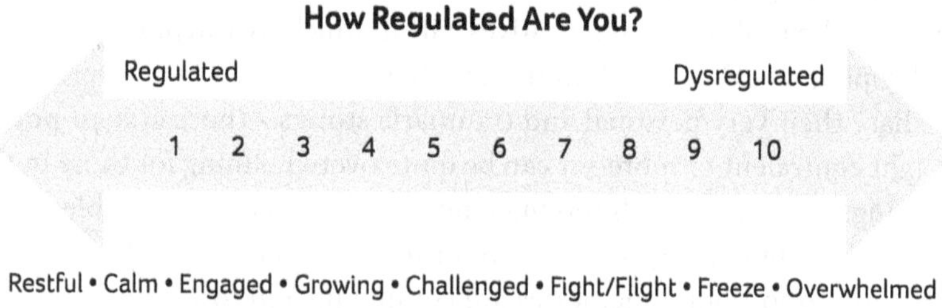

How Regulated Are You?

Regulated ← 1 2 3 4 5 6 7 8 9 10 → Dysregulated

Restful • Calm • Engaged • Growing • Challenged • Fight/Flight • Freeze • Overwhelmed

FIGURE 3.1 NERVOUS SYSTEM SELF-REGULATION SCALE

> **Journal Prompt.** Take a moment. Ground your feet and sitting bones. Place a hand on your belly and a hand on your heart. Don't try to change anything. Scan your body for overall activation. Then answer the questions below:
>
> - How activated are you (using a number on the scale)? How do you know this? What did you notice?
> - What direction were you headed (more or less activated)?
> - How do you know this? What did you notice?

PREPAREDNESS—RESOURCE, ASSESS, PAUSE, DE-ESCALATE, AND CONNECT

Knowing your number and assessing the potential number of your students allows you to select practices to facilitate movement to or stability within a more regulated state. This is attunement. For example, you can use more calming and grounding practice for higher numbers, and activating practices for lower numbers. As you will learn in this book, these numbers are associated with specific states of the nervous system, very relevant to trauma and trauma symptoms.

TIR PRACTICE: GROUND, BREATHE, AND ORIENT

It is important to have a few accessible ways to self-regulate you and/or your students. Ground, breathe, and orient is an excellent practice that helps stop escalation to higher levels of activation and can serve to lower activation levels. This process has three simple steps:

- increase connection to the earth (groundedness)
- focus on slowing the breath
- decrease input of visual stimuli (orientation).

For yourself, you can move to a more grounded position, such as a Mountain Pose, or a seated posture in a chair, grounding your feet and sitting bones, slowly regulating your breath, and gazing at something steady in front of you. For your students, this might include cueing your students to take a Child's Pose (facing toward the floor, knees bent, folding at the hips, head toward the mat, arms outstretched or by the side body) or Crocodile Pose (lying face down, forearms folded over one another, forehead on forearms) and then instructing them to take slow, subtle breaths and soften their eyes. The goal is to provide support (groundedness), calm the nervous system (slow, subtle breaths), and decrease activation (orient, decrease, or soften the gaze).

> **Journal Prompt.** What are some different ways you might implement the ground, breathe, and orient technique? Experiment with a few grounding poses assessing yourself on the self-regulation scale and record your before and after ratings next to each pose practice.

> **PRACTICING THE PAUSE**
> Any time, any place, and for any reason, you can always PAUSE. Pause = stop what you are doing, A = assess how you are and what you need, and USE = use your resources.

Trauma-Informed Practice: The PAUSE

Practicing the PAUSE is helpful when you (or a student) are feeling quite dysregulated—around a 6, 7, or 8 on the self-regulation scale. When using this for yourself, simply take a break from what you are doing and follow the steps. If you are teaching this to a student, do so in a one-on-one situation. The PAUSE is also a three-step process (Cook-Cottone, 2023):

- **Step 1—Pause:** Stop what you are doing. Press your feet into the ground below you and take four gentle breaths.
- **Step 2—Assess:** Assess how you are doing. Take a moment and scan your body. Do you feel activated, anxious, or stressed? What is your number on the self-regulation scale? Is it 5 or above? Is it a good time to take a break and use your resources?
- **Step 3—Use your resources:** Implement the resources you might need. These can include the following:
  - Reaching out to a good friend, the trainer for your yoga teacher training, your therapist, or trusted family member if your levels of distress are high.
  - Turn toward one or more of your inner resources.
  - See the "My Resources" section of your journal and choose a practice that you know will be helpful.
  - You might engage in one of the calming or balancing practices described in this book.
  - If you feel some distress and are able to self-regulate on your own, perhaps you just need to take a break and focus on something else for a while.

You can get back to this work (or any other work) when *you* are ready (Cook-Cottone, 2023). Throughout this book, we will be offering you reminders to PAUSE.

PREPAREDNESS—RESOURCE, ASSESS, PAUSE, DE-ESCALATE, AND CONNECT

Journal Prompt. Describe a situation in which you think it might be helpful for you to practice the PAUSE. If you think back, what might your score have been on the self-regulation scale? What support or resources could you turn to? Going forward, what score on the self-regulation scale is a good signal for taking a PAUSE?

TIR PRINCIPLE: SOMETIMES JUST BREATHING TOGETHER IS ENOUGH
Intentional, gentle, and slow breathing can help down-regulate a dysregulated nervous system.

TIR PRACTICE: BREATHE-WITH
I (CCC) learned the Breathe-With practice at a Yoga Service Council gathering with Sue Jones, a trauma-informed yoga expert. It is simple and very powerful. It is a form of peer support. If someone in the group shares and appears to become dysregulated (e.g., breath dysregulated, crying), anyone in the group can say, "If it's okay, let's breathe with [person's name]." The person who called for the Breathe-With begins and guides the group through the breathwork. This includes a reminder to ground the body, engage the core, and orient toward the breath. Then, the leader guides a cycle of three intentional, gentle, and slow breaths: "Breathe in [pause], and breathe out [pause], breathe in [pause], and breathe out [pause], breathe in [pause], and breathe out [pause]."

This practice tends to calm, or down-regulate, the whole group and gives space for the person who has become dysregulated to self-regulate. If it seems appropriate, the cycle can be repeated. Note that it can be very helpful to introduce this concept and practice as a group before it is necessary.

TIR PRINCIPLE: KNOW A DE-ESCALATION PROTOCOL
Yoga teachers should know and be prepared to implement a de-escalation protocol—recognize, stabilize, and refer.

TIR PRACTICE: DE-ESCALATION PROTOCOL—RECOGNIZE, STABILIZE, AND REFER

A de-escalation protocol is to be used when a student in class (or in your teacher training) becomes very activated and overwhelmed, and needs immediate support. This would look like a 7–10 on the self-regulation scale or someone who is quickly escalating from a lower number to a higher number.

> I (CCC) was conducting trauma-informed training several years ago. A student (they/them) shared a very detailed description of trauma they had experienced (it was about a 100-pound weight share). I don't think they intended to share their past trauma at that level; however, as they did, it was clear they were unraveling. We took several breaths together (see the Breathe-With practice above). The class seemed regulated, as did the person who shared. The session ended and it was late. Another student (she/her) came to me as the rest of the students were leaving. She began to tell me that a lot had come up for them during the share; however, as she spoke, she became incapacitated. She couldn't talk. There were tears coming down her face, and she lost eye contact with me. Her breath became dysregulated and short and choppy. She appeared to be moving into a panic response. I engaged in the de-escalation protocol described here. After about ten minutes of us co-regulating, she was able to calmly and effectively describe her experience to me. Her nervous system was likely at around a 5 (coming down from an 8 or 9) and she was able to speak to me, including eye contact and an even and steady breath. This is the exact type of situation within which you can use this de-escalation protocol.

Step One: Recognize (and Assess)

- The first step is to notice that your student is stressed or showing signs of trauma. Be sure that you know the signs (see Chapter 2).
- Assess the moment. Is anyone in danger or hurt? Do you need to call 911? Do you need more help? Should someone cover the class or space so you can support the student?
- Take action if you answer yes to any of those questions.

Step Two (Basic Steps): Stabilize

- The second step is to support the student so they can feel more grounded and stable.

PREPAREDNESS—RESOURCE, ASSESS, PAUSE, DE-ESCALATE, AND CONNECT

- Student stays in class (or public setting):
  - In class, move discreetly toward the student and directly ask, "Are you okay?" and/or "Is there anything you need right now?"
  - You can also simply be with the student—do nothing. Stand in close proximity, offer a comforting assist/tissue, and give space. Be a model for allowing and welcoming all emotions and experiences (if appropriate in current setting).
  - If the student's behavior is disruptive to the class, or the class or setting does not seem sufficiently private for stabilizing, take the student to a hallway, office, or another private setting. Say, "Let's go to my office [or other private location] and take a break."
  - If you leave the class, ask a fellow teacher to cover or invite the class to take ten minutes to rest or practice independently.
- Student is in a private setting (or needs more support than you can offer the class or in a public setting):
  - Offer them a seat.
  - Align yourself to be at the same height or slightly lower than the student and well grounded (kneel down, take a seat next to them).
  - Soften your eyes, your shoulders. Work to be grounded and steady. This will be potentially calming for the student's nervous system.
  - Directly ask, "Are you okay?" and/or "Is there anything you need right now?"
  - You can also simply be with the student, doing nothing, just holding a comforting space.
  - Ask "Can I place my hand on your shoulder or back?" if that feels like something they might need. Make sure this is culturally appropriate in regard to gender, student/teacher relationships, and school/studio/hospital policy.
  - If yes, place your hand on their shoulder or on their back, behind their heart—no lower than the shoulder blades. Palms flat, fingers together as an extension of the palms.
  - Match your breath rate to theirs and then slow your breath rate with them. You can verbalize this: "I am breathing too. I am going to slow down my breathing a little bit at a time to help my body feel more calm. Let's try this together." Engage in gentle, slow breaths.
  - To yourself (silently), say a mantra, the loving-kindness meditation ("May you be happy. May you be well. May you be peaceful and at ease"). This will help slow and center your thoughts and presence and create a more calming presence.

- You can offer a tissue—do this as support, not as a cue that crying is not accepted here: "This is for supporting, not stopping tears (or crying)."

Step Two (Advanced Steps): Grounding, Orienting, and Resourcing

- If the student is very upset, seems to be having a reaction or trauma response, or is dissociated (seeming as if they are not mentally present), continue the being-with practices and then engage in a Grounding, Orienting, and Resourcing protocol.
- Grounding, Orienting, and Resourcing is a step-by-step process for getting your student back to the here and now, connecting or reconnecting to their yoga practice, and is good to use when someone has been distracted or triggered.
- *Grounding* is reconnecting to the earth/ground below you and your own body. You can guide the yoga student through the process using this script:
  - Press your feet into the floor, place your hands on your belly and/or on your belly and your heart.
  - Breathe. Breathe into your hands.
  - Press your feet into the floor (and maybe your sit bones into your chair or cushion). Push one foot and then the other into the floor.
  - Soften—do not lock—your knees.
  - Engage the muscles in your legs and your core, and gently release and repeat a few times.
  - With your hands on your belly and heart, breathe.
  - *Be with and breathe with your yoga student:* "Try breathing with me. Breathe in 1, 2, 3, and breathe out 1, 2, 3, 4." Repeat this several times, slowing a bit each time.
  - Grounding helps you feel connected to earth, have an awareness of and connection to your own body, and adds a sensation of being centered.
- *Orienting* is the process of getting to this moment, in this space, in your body. Orienting builds on the grounding practice above. You can guide the student through the process of orienting by using this script.
  - Build on your grounding work. Connect to the earth, your body, and your breath.
  - You are right here, right now.
  - To become further oriented, survey (look around) the room,

PREPAREDNESS—RESOURCE, ASSESS, PAUSE, DE-ESCALATE, AND CONNECT

   notice other people, items (yoga mats, blocks), and get a good sense of what is happening around you. Breathe.
  - Next, find your space. Notice the edges of your mat and draw your awareness into where your body and the mat meet [if they are in class; if not, ask them to notice something specific, the details of it].
  - Press your hands or feet into your mat (the bench, the floor).
  - Next, turn back inward to your body. Feel your body as it connects to the earth and breathe.
  - You might even say to yourself, "I am here, in my yoga space, on my yoga mat, pressing my hands and/or feet into my mat." You can also say this with them.
  - If they are struggling, say, "It might be helpful to tell me *five* things you see around you" [pause for their answer].
  - "Tell me *four* things you can touch around you" [pause for their answer].
  - "Tell me *three* things you can hear" [pause for their answer].
  - "Tell me *two* things you can smell" [pause for their answer].
  - Optional: "Tell me *one* thing you can taste" [pause for their answer]. Adaptation: "Tell me one thing, right now, you know to be true. For example, mine is that I love my dog."
- *Resourcing* is the process of connecting to inner resources.
  - Your inner resources are anything that helps you connect to your sense of wellbeing. Inner resources can include the grounding and orienting work listed above.
  - You can help the student connect to their inner resources by using this script: "You might have a dear friend, family member, a special place, or a pet that you can call to mind that reminds you that you are okay. Can you think about something like that now? Can you tell me about it?"
  - You can also consider offering affirmations like "I am worth the effort" or another mantra that helps you feel okay such as "I can feel my feelings and be okay" or "I know how to calm myself when I am triggered or upset." "Is there a saying that helps you feel just a little more calm? Can you tell me?"

Step Three: Refer

- In the moment, be sure you have followed through with each of the sections in:

TRAUMA-INFORMED AND TRAUMA-RESPONSIVE YOGA TEACHING

- Step One: Recognize
- Step Two: Stabilize (basic and advanced).
- Know that it is okay for the student to have their experience. Allow it to be what it needs to be for the student. You are not expected to fix anything—the goal here is to notice something is happening (recognize) and then support the student (stabilize).
- Refer the student to someone that can support their healing/recovery/treatment.
- Make sure you have a list of the local counselors or therapists in your area that work with PTSD. This is the list you can offer to students who may need a referral.
- Ask your student to tell you who they might go to for support. Suggest a stable and safe family member, a person from their church, a counselor or therapist, their doctor, etc.
- Document the experience, your actions, and the referrals. Report to your adviser, program leader, or studio owner.

DE-ESCALATION PROTOCOL CUE CARD

1. Recognize and Assess
2. Stabilize (Basic Steps) and Grounding, Orienting, and Resourcing (Advanced Steps)
3. Refer

Journal Prompt. Practice the de-escalation protocol with a friend or classmate. Take turns being the yoga teacher and the yoga student. What parts were the most challenging as a teacher? Which parts were the most soothing and grounding as a student? List the situations within the space that you teach and practice for which the de-escalation protocol might be helpful.

TIR PRACTICE: CONNECTION—DO YOUR STUDENTS KNOW HOW TO ASK FOR HELP?

As we close this chapter, we ask some final questions about connection. Do you notice that students do ask for help? How do they do this? Do

PREPAREDNESS—RESOURCE, ASSESS, PAUSE, DE-ESCALATE, AND CONNECT

your students know how to ask for help? Does your space feel open and accepting enough for students to ask for help? Contemplate this question as you move and teach in your studio or space. Note that the lack of questions or requests for support may mean that students do not feel they can ask or that they don't have access to a way in which they feel they can ask. Being trauma-informed means you are making sure those who need support know how and have a way to ask for it. If a method is not there, create one.

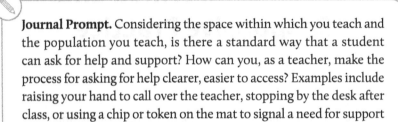

Journal Prompt. Considering the space within which you teach and the population you teach, is there a standard way that a student can ask for help and support? How can you, as a teacher, make the process for asking for help clearer, easier to access? Examples include raising your hand to call over the teacher, stopping by the desk after class, or using a chip or token on the mat to signal a need for support or assistance.

TEACHER TRAINING DISCUSSION QUESTIONS

1. What does it mean to share using the five-pound weight guideline? Why is this important?

2. Name and describe some ways you might use the self-regulation scale.

3. Describe the Breathe-With technique and when it might be helpful.

4. What are some signs it might be a good time for you to practice the PAUSE? What might you notice physiologically, emotionally, and cognitively (your thoughts and words)?

5. Describe your experience practicing the de-escalation protocol.

6. Explain how you can verify that students who attend your yoga classes, studio, or yoga space know that they can ask for help or support.

CHAPTER 4

Mindful Self-Care as a Trauma-Informed and Responsive Practice

sa tu dîrgha-kâla-nairantarya-satkârâsevito dëëha-bhûmiï

Yoga Sutra I:14

This [practice] becomes a firm resting-place, when followed long, persistently, with earnestness.

Charles Johnston (1912)

Consider the quote attributed to Rumi, a 13th-century Persian poet: "Wherever you go, be the soul of that place." As yoga teachers, we aspire to embody that kind of presence. Yoga is a soulful practice, built on a foundation of mindful self-care. Students enter the yoga space needing and wanting inspiration, kindness, and a love of the practice. The teacher can be a barrier, and perhaps even harmful, when they enter the yoga space stressed out, burnt out, without personal practice, and perhaps detached from why they began teaching in the first place.

Mindful self-care is comprehensive. It serves to support the trauma-informed values of safety, trustworthiness, mutuality, and empowerment. It includes knowing and honoring your scope of practice and developing solid professional boundaries, while also developing and maintaining your personal yoga practice and daily mindful self-care. It includes creating and maintaining a manageable teaching schedule, ongoing professional development and supervision, and knowing when to get help. This chapter will review each of these aspects of yoga teacher self-care and will end with remembering your why ("I began teaching yoga because...").

Prioritizing your own self-care demonstrates the level to which you value it. It can be so easy to discount self-care as something indulgent or adjunct—our culture does that. However, as Dan Siegel writes below, a deeply mindful and intentional practice of self-care is critical to how well we negotiate the future of our personal and collective wellbeing.

> Because no matter the challenges we confront... There is no escaping this reality, no matter what others, or we, try to say about it. If we don't care for ourselves, we'll be limited in how we can care for others. It is that simple. And it is that important—for you, for others, and for our planet. (Siegel, 2010, p. 3)

TIR PRINCIPLE: THE MORE YOU CARE, THE MORE YOU NEED SELF-CARE
Those who care the most are at the highest risk for burnout and compassion fatigue. The need for self-care is even higher for those who care a lot.

Burnout and Compassion Fatigue

Those who care the most are believed to be at the highest risk for burnout. This may be due to a phenomenon called *compassion fatigue*. Compassion fatigue is a term coined by psychologist Charles R. Figley, PhD, founder of the Traumatology Institute at Tulane University (Clay, 2022). It occurs when you take in the suffering of your clients who have experienced or are experiencing extreme stress or trauma (Clay, 2022). Figley characterizes compassion fatigue as an occupational hazard of any professional who uses their heart. Its symptoms are aligned with those of burnout, including loss of productivity, depression, intrusive thoughts, jumpiness, fatigue, feeling on the edge or trapped, and difficulty separating professional and personal life (Clay, 2022).

TIR PRACTICE: ASSESSMENT—ARE YOU AT RISK FOR BURNOUT OR COMPASSION FATIGUE?

It is important to take a pause from time to time to consider whether or not you are suffering from burnout, need to take a break, or are in need of additional supervision and/or support. Take a few minutes and answer the questions below.

TRAUMA-INFORMED AND TRAUMA-RESPONSIVE YOGA TEACHING

1. Do you feel rundown, tired, and/or drained?
2. Are you having trouble getting prepared for teaching class, showing up on time, delivering class, and/or taking care of your yoga teaching responsibilities?
3. Have you shown up for a class impaired and/or self-medicated?
4. Have you stopped practicing yoga and mindfulness regularly?
5. Do you have frequent negative thoughts about teaching yoga, the yoga students, and/or your yoga studio or organization?
6. Do you have difficulty empathizing with, feeling kind towards, and/or supporting your yoga students and/or fellow yoga teachers?
7. Do you feel unmotivated to teach your yoga classes?
8. Do you frequently sub-out your classes?
9. Are you easily irritated by the yoga students, your studio or organization, and/or your fellow teachers?
10. Do you feel stuck, trapped, and/or overwhelmed?
11. Are you not having fun doing the things that used to make you happy?
12. Do you feel avoidant of and/or resistant toward your personal practice?
13. Did you stop feeling excited about yoga?
14. Do you feel that you are no longer getting what you wanted or needed from your yoga teaching experience?
15. Do you remember why you wanted to teach yoga?

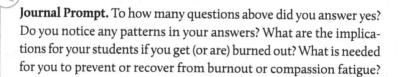

Journal Prompt. To how many questions above did you answer yes? Do you notice any patterns in your answers? What are the implications for your students if you get (or are) burned out? What is needed for you to prevent or recover from burnout or compassion fatigue?

It's okay if you answered yes to some or all of those questions. Knowledge and awareness foster empowerment. When I (CCC) am working as a psychologist, I will sometimes have a patient ask me if someone they love will ever change (e.g., quit drinking, start taking care of themselves, etc.). My answer is always the same: "Maybe. Given supportive environmental factors, it comes down to awareness, willingness, and work." By asking ourselves the hard questions about our relationship with our yoga teaching and practice, we are digging into the first requirement for change: awareness. We can't change something about which we are not aware. The next step is looking at willingness. Given that you have bought and are reading this book, it is my guess that you have a certain amount of willingness, and this is a good sign. Last is the work. The rest of this chapter will take you through the important aspects of taking care of yourself as a yoga teacher (i.e., the work). These important practices will help you prevent burnout and keep you (or get you back) on track to being excited about sharing your yoga practice and knowledge with your students.

TIR PRINCIPLE: SCOPE OF PRACTICE
Teach within your scope of practice.

TIR PRACTICE: HONORING SCOPE OF PRACTICE
Being clear about what is and what is not your job is central to mindful self-care. Very simply put, yoga teachers teach yoga. Yoga is an ancient system of physical, mental, and spiritual practices that help the practitioner achieve a state of unity of body and mind, such as yoga philosophy, asana (postures), pranayama (breathwork), relaxation, mantras, meditation, seva (service), and self-study (Cook-Cottone, 2015; Yoga Alliance, 2020b).

It is stressful for you, potentially harmful for your students, and a legal risk when you practice outside of your competencies. Defining the scope of practice of a yoga teacher helps us clarify what is and is not our job/role. Yoga practice, as delivered by a yoga teacher, is not a treatment. A yoga teacher (unless otherwise trained and licensed) is *not* a medical doctor, nutritionist, physical therapist, mental health counselor, psychologist, psychiatrist, marriage and family therapist, occupational therapist, or substance use counselor. Each of those professions takes anywhere from four to 12+ years of post-high school education and state licensure. A 200-, 300-, or even 500-hour yoga teacher certification would not be sufficient to engage in professional activities in any of those fields.

In 2020, Yoga Alliance published its first guidance on scope of practice specifically defining the role of a yoga teacher and advising yoga teachers to only teach within their permitted scope:

> [Yoga teachers are allowed] to teach yoga and to offer instruction and education on yoga practices and principles that responsibly reflect the level of yoga education, training, and experience of both the [yoga teachers] and

the [yoga student(s)]. [Yoga teachers] may teach yoga in a group, in a one-on-one setting, or online. [Yoga teachers] must limit teaching to practices and learnings that align with yoga philosophy and the lineage, style, and methodology for which the [yoga teacher] is qualified and in accordance with the competencies described in the Yoga Alliance Common Core Curriculum Standards. (Yoga Alliance, 2020b, p. 4)

Use your urges or desires to act outside of your scope of practice to guide your professional development. For example, if you are interested in offering nutritional advice, perhaps this is an indication that you'd like to go into the field of nutrition and it's time to continue your education and become a dietician. If you feel yourself pulled to interact with students about their mental health struggles and treatment, this may be an indication that you would like to go into the mental health field. If you feel yourself drawn to the more therapeutic aspects of yoga, consider training to become a certified yoga therapist. According to the International Association of Yoga Therapists (IAYT), "Yoga therapy is the professional application of the principles and practices of yoga to promote health and well-being within a therapeutic relationship that includes personalized assessment, goal setting, lifestyle management, and yoga practices for individuals or small groups" (IAYT, n.d.).

> **TIR PRINCIPLE: PROFESSIONAL BOUNDARIES**
> Keeping professional boundaries is good for you and your yoga students.

TIR PRACTICE: KEEP PROFESSIONAL BOUNDARIES

Conceptually, scope of practice can seem quite clear. In practice, however, it can get a little complicated. When a student confides in you, it is good to immediately explain the scope of your training and make a referral. Each time you talk to a student about issues in an area in which you are not trained, you may be delaying care from those trained to help them. In this way, by not setting a boundary, you are delaying their care.

- "That sounds so overwhelming. I'm not trained in [the areas in which they are struggling]. I know a few really good therapists in the area who could be helpful and supportive. Here are their cards. I'm here for your yoga and that can help with your stress."

- "I know Dr. Smith (she/her). She loves yoga too and she is a specialist in eating disorders. Here is her card."
- "Dr. Grant (they/them) is a wonderful physical therapist. Here is their card. They specialize in shoulders and shoulder injuries. As for yoga, take it easy during x, y, and z poses in class and take a break whenever you feel you need one. If you are in pain, you might want to hold off until you get medical clearance."

Your city, town, or village likely has a healing community filled with professionals and specialists trained to help, treat, and support your yoga students. By making effective referrals, you are partnering with the healing community. Take time to get to know the professionals in your area. Look for psychologists, social workers, mental health professionals, physical therapists, occupational therapists, medical doctors, and nutritionists who also practice or teach. They are great referrals for your yoga students. If you offer teacher training, commission local professionals to teach segments of your curriculum to deepen these relationships and model these connections to your trainees. These same professionals will, in turn, learn to trust you for knowing and honoring scope of practice, and refer their clients to you. If you are from a small town or your yoga sessions are in an area without access, this will be more challenging. Connect with the other service organizations and the primary care physicians in your area to make sure you can provide accessible referrals for your students.

Consider this scenario:

> You just finished offering a class with a theme of Maitri, or self-love. The class went well and you have a good feeling about how it was experienced by the students. As the students leave, many are thanking you and smiling, communicating overall positive feelings. You notice that one student (she/her) is lingering. She waits until everyone else has left and begins to talk to you about her current experiences with domestic violence. You get a sense she is in a terrible situation and that this is far outside of your scope of practice. You are not sure how to advise her. You listen and encourage her to get support and offer her a few cards of local therapists and clinics that you know are effective, offer sliding scale fees, and have openings. The next class, she stays after again, this time telling you more and staying after for almost 25 minutes. The next class, she stays again, this time for 20 minutes, and the content is quite serious. You refer her to a domestic violence shelter, giving her their emergency number and contact. For the fourth class in a row, she stays after. This time she stayed for 30 minutes. You encourage her to

reach out to one of the therapists to which you referred her, and she jokes, "I don't need a therapist—I have you."

Journal Prompt. Consider these questions:

1. At what point does a student begin to see you, the yoga teacher, as their therapist? What are the warning signs as presented in the scenario above?
2. How can you more clearly communicate to the student that you are not trained to support her and more effectively encourage her to seek professional support?
3. What is at risk here if the student believes that the yoga teacher is her therapeutic support system?
4. What might it feel like as the yoga teacher to have this additional work (20 to 30 minutes of supportive counseling) added to the work of teaching a yoga class?

Developing and Maintaining Your Personal Yoga Practice

There is a Latin phrase reflecting the power of a personal practice: *nemo dat quod non habet*. It means, we cannot give what we do not have. It is an old legal term referring to the selling of another person's property—if it is not your boat, you cannot sell it or give it away. Consider this: you cannot deliver a yoga class that is attuned, sensitive, and responsive for other people's bodies if you do not practice yoga that is attuned, sensitive, and responsive in your own body.

> **TIR PRINCIPLE:** NEMO DAT QUOD NON HABET
> You cannot give what you do not have.

The most effective yoga teachers have a dedicated yoga practice. Teaching yoga is not doing yoga (as in having your own practice). Yes, we do mean practice for practice's sake. Patanjali reinforces this premise in yoga sutra I:14: "Practice becomes firmly grounded when well attended to for a long time without break and in all earnestness" (Satchidananda, 1985, p. 6).

> **TIR PRINCIPLE: PRACTICE IS EVERYTHING**
> Your personal practice will be the foundation of your trauma-informed and responsive yoga teaching.

It is in the regular practice of yoga that you can start to really notice your body's *response* to practice. As you practice, your awareness and understanding will begin to unfold. In the early years of practice, it is common for both practice and teaching to focus on asana—the poses. As you know, it takes a lot of effort to learn the poses, the alignment of the pose, and the words to use to cue the pose. It takes time and study to fully understand how and why the mechanisms of a pose work—this comes much later. For example, it can take several years of practice and teaching to learn how to link your breath and movement, and even longer to integrate what you are learning and feeling into your whole body. JS put it this way:

> Because I thought I understood how breathing affected my nervous system, I simply intellectualized the information, meaning I stored it away somewhere in the "got it, don't need it right now" folder in my memory. The conversation in my head went something like this: focus on how to correctly place your feet and arms in Warrior Pose 2, breathing you already know about. And I would inadvertently tune out the teaching I was receiving about breathing, the rationale being that since I was breathing, I assumed I knew all about breathing. In reality, I knew barely nothing about breathing. But I didn't yet know that I didn't know.

Over time, you will develop an embodied awareness of your nervous system responses to each pose and breath. This grants you an increased awareness of your students' experience and an ability to safely and effectively guide them through their own process of awareness, understanding, and choice.

How Frequently Should You Practice?

Habits drive behavior. When we repeat the same action again and again, our brain creates neural pathways through a process called neuroplasticity (Spence, 2021). Generally speaking, you should integrate practices such as meditation and relaxation every day (Ross *et al.*, 2012). For example, you could begin with 2–10 minutes of meditation and listen to a relaxation or sleep-enhancing relaxation audio at night. You can build this up or keep a steady daily practice at exactly that duration. Research has shown that frequent asana practice (around three times per week) can be beneficial (Cook-Cottone, 2013). Asana practice can be every day if varied in intensity and form. Variations should be based on what the body needs and not on adherence to a rigid schedule or practice goals. For some, vinyasa practice might make sense for your nervous system every other day with yin practices and other physical activity interwoven (e.g., walking, running, and fun interactive sports like tennis and pickleball).

Journal Prompt. Table 4.1 is a sample chart for planning and recording your daily practice. At the beginning of the week, plan out your practices. At the end of the week, jot down what you notice.

TIR PRACTICE: DAILY MINDFUL SELF-CARE

Mindful self-care is a construct first coined by Dr. Catherine Cook-Cottone (one of the authors of this book) and Dr. Wendy Guyker (she/her), researchers from the University at Buffalo, State University of New York. In 2018, they published the Mindful Self-Care Scale, which is a scientifically developed scale used to assess and research mindful self-care. There is a substantial body of work studying the Mindful Self-Care Scale (more than 150 studies). To access the article search "Mindful Self-Care Scale" (Cook-Cottone & Guyker, 2018) in Google Scholar. Research on mindful self-care indicates that steady and intentional practice of self-care is protective, preventing the onset of mental health symptoms and burnout. It has also been found to increase wellbeing, positive body image, and a positive outlook on life, and to decrease addictive and self-destructive behaviors (Cook-Cottone, 2015, 2017; Cook-Cottone et al., 2019; Cook-Cottone & Guyker, 2018).

Mindful self-care is defined as the daily process of being aware of and attending to one's basic physiological and emotional needs, including the shaping of one's daily routine, relationships, and environment as needed to promote self-care (Cook-Cottone, 2015, 2017; Cook-Cottone et al., 2019). It is not the marketed, branded version of self-care that depicts privileged individuals getting a massage at a spa with cucumber slices over their eyes and in their glass of water. Although that does sound nice! Mindful self-care is a mindful, day-to-day practice that creates the experience of positive embodiment, living in and through the body in ways that create and maintain wellbeing (Cook-Cottone, 2023). You can take the 33-item

Table 4.1 Developing My Practice Plan

Practice	Sunday	Monday	Tuesday	Wednesday	Thursday	Friday	Saturday
Meditation							
Relaxation							
Asana							
Breathwork							
Study							
Seva							
How did your practice feel this week? What did you notice? What adjustments would you like to make for next week?							

online version of the scale at https://ed.buffalo.edu/mindful-assessment.html. You will be emailed your results with associated recommendations. You can find the other 84-item and the 33-item versions of the scale at www.catherinecookcottone.com; these can be printed and used for free. I (CCC) use the longer version in yoga teacher training and for courses on self-care for mental health professionals. Table 4.2 covers a few of the mindful self-care practices that you can practice in each domain.

Table 4.2 The Ten Domains of Mindful Self-Care and Associated Practices

Mindful Self-Care Domain	Mindful Self-Care Practices (three examples for each domain)
Nutrition and Hydration	• Drink at least 6–8 cups of water daily • Adjust water intake for exercise and exertion • Eat a variety of nutritious foods
Exercise	• Exercise (move) 30–60 minutes per day • Engage in fun physical activities such as games, dancing, and jumping in leaves • Plan and schedule your exercise for the week
Rest	• Sleep enough each night to feel rested and restored when you awaken • Take rest when needed (e.g., when not feeling well, after a long run) • Plan and schedule pleasant activities unrelated to work or school
Physical and Medical Care	• Engage in medical and dental care to prevent and treat illness and disease • Refrain from (or decrease) smoking tobacco, taking recreational drugs, and drinking alcohol • Practice overall cleanliness and hygiene
Self-Soothing	• Use subtle and deep breathing to relax • Listen to relax (e.g., music, podcast, relaxation script, rainforest sounds) • Seek out touch to relax (e.g., pet an animal, cuddle a soft blanket, float in a pool, put on comfy clothes)
Self-Compassion	• Notice, without judgment, when you are struggling (e.g., feeling resistance, falling short of your goals, not completing as much as you'd like) • Refrain from punitively and harshly judging your progress and effort • Give yourself permission to feel your feelings (e.g., allow yourself to cry)

Relationships	• Spend time with people who are good to you (e.g., support, encourage, and believe in you) • Spend time around people who would respect your choice if you said "No" • Make sure you can easily identify someone who would listen to you if you become upset (e.g., a close friend, counselor, group)
Environmental Factors	• Maintain a manageable schedule • Maintain a comforting and pleasing living environment • Keep your work or school area organized to support your work or school tasks
Spiritual Practice	• Explore ways to find meaning or a larger purpose in your private and personal life (e.g., seva, doing something for a cause) • Spend time in a spiritual place (e.g., nature, church, meditation room) • Spend time doing something you hope will make a positive difference in the world (e.g., volunteer at a soup kitchen, take time to care for someone else)
Self-Awareness and Mindfulness	• Practice having a calm awareness of your thoughts, feelings, and body • Carefully and intentionally select which of your thoughts and feelings you will use to guide your actions • Meditate in some form (e.g., sitting, walking, prayer)
General	• Engage in a variety of mindful self-care strategies and practices • Plan your mindful self-care • Consistently explore new ways of bringing self-care into your life

(Cook-Cottone & Guyker, 2018)

TIR PRACTICE: EMBODYING YOUR MINDFUL SELF-CARE—ARTFUL SELF-CARE

Mindful self-care is not quite as simple as going through an assessment or checklist and doing a few things each day—although that is not a bad way to start! As you begin to explore the impact of self-care on your life, you will begin realizing it can be a nuanced or *artful* process (Cook-Cottone, 2023). As you develop your self-care plan, address these areas: A—Attuned, R—Responsive, T—Taking action, F—Fun, U—Union, and L—Loving-kindness.

A—Attuned. While generally adding mindful self-care practice to your daily routine will help reduce stress and enhance wellbeing, your mindful self-care is most effective when it is attuned to what you need.

> **Journal Prompt.** Look through this chapter and take a moment to pause and scan your body, asking, "Body, what do you need? Heart, what do you need? Mind, what do you need?" What needs are present for you right now?

R—Responsive. Humans have fundamental needs to be seen and heard. Mindful self-care is one way to show your body, heart, and mind they are seen and heard. Notice what you need within these three aspects of self and select mindful self-care behaviors serving those specific needs. In this way, you are seeing and listening to yourself in a way you will feel deeply as you practice.

> **Journal Prompt.** Take a look at the needs you expressed above and the list of mindful self-care behaviors. What mindful self-care actions will be most responsive to your needs in the present moment?

T—Taking action. Mindful self-care is much easier to plan than to actually implement daily. Taking action means putting your mindful self-care plan to work! Ask yourself, "Did I engage in the self-care that I know I need?" Taking action is supported by planning and scheduling your self-care. Ultimately, it is in the doing that you will experience the results.

> **Journal Prompt.** Go back to your practice schedule and add in your mindful self-care as a non-negotiable. Schedule a specific place and time for the mindful self-care practices that take dedicated time (formal practices) and then make a note of the mindful practices you can weave into your day (informal practices) such as listening to music while you work, noticing your thoughts, and pausing to take short breaks hourly.

F—Fun. We can all get very serious when exploring topics like trauma or our mindful self-care practices. It turns out that those who have fun taking care of themselves and engaging in meaningful work have the greatest sustainability. If you are serious about your mindful self-care, you will need to ensure you are having some fun!

MINDFUL SELF-CARE AS A TRAUMA-INFORMED AND RESPONSIVE PRACTICE

Journal Prompt. When you look over your mindful self-care plan, does any of it look fun? If your answer is yes, great, list what looks fun here. If your answer is no, pause and look through the lists, consider what is available in your area, reach out to some friends, and add in a few things each week that are fun!

U—Union. The foundational model for yoga is union of body and mind. The mindful self-care practices you choose will be most effective if they facilitate body and mind integration. For example, if you choose exercise and run many miles every day, disconnecting from your body and running through pain, this is not mindful self-care. The end result is a separation of body and mind, or mind over matter (your body). Instead, if you choose running, perhaps run for 45 minutes three times a week, selecting a different park or nature trail for your run. Another option is alternating running and yoga classes, or pausing during your run to take a meditation break. The goal is to consider how you can cultivate the mind-body connection during our mindful self-care practice.

Journal Prompt. While reflecting on your mindful self-care plan and your past behaviors, do you notice any behaviors in which you tend to check out or dissociate? Push yourself too hard or to injury? In what ways can you cultivate the integration of mind and body in your mindful self-care practices?

TIR PRINCIPLE: MINDFUL SELF-CARE IS A GENEROUS ACT
Engaging in mindful self-care is something that benefits both you and the people in your life. You become the best version of yourself for you and them.

L—Loving-kindness. When practiced effectively and with loving-kindness, mindful self-care can enhance your relationships and support others. Mindful self-care is actually one of the most generous things you can do. I (CCC) always ask my psychologist in training if they know of a family member or friend who does not take care of themselves. Most do. Then I ask, "Wouldn't it be incredibly generous for them to engage in self-care?" Across the board, students agree. When someone does not take care of themselves, others suffer. Those who do not engage in self-care can be bitter, edgy, difficult to be around, and, in fact, cause others to need to do work (e.g., take them to doctor appointments because they smoked for 40 years and now suffer the consequence, worry because they drink daily and are late on rent). In this way, self-care is a very generous and loving act.

> **TIR PRINCIPLE:** MINDFUL SELF-CARE IS COLLECTIVE CARE
> Your mindful self-care should serve, and not interfere with, others' mindful self-care.

There is another aspect of self-care that is important to highlight. Self-care is not selfish behavior. Self-care plans should always take into account the impact on others. Consider this scenario:

> Janice (she/her) is part of a not-for-profit group that holds events to raise money to pay yoga teachers to offer classes in hospitals, domestic violence shelters, and community centers. She is on the current event committee and takes on several substantial tasks—securing the tables and chairs, driving gear and sale items to the venue, and leading the set-up and break-down team. On the night before the event, she reaches out to the other committee members to express that her involvement on the event committee has been too stressful and she must back out of her responsibilities the following day, in service of her own self-care. She is sorry, but this is something she must do.

Journal Prompt. Where did Janice's mindful self-care first begin to break down? In what ways did she use the concept of self-care that caused extra work and stress for her other committee members? In what ways did Janice's behavior not integrate loving-kindness for herself or others? How could Janice have engaged in self-care in ways that would have also been acts of collective care for her other committee members?

TIR PRACTICE: A MINDFUL AND COLLECTIVE CARE MEDITATION

The ARTFUL path to mindful self-care holds that you are also engaged in collective care. It is not an either or, me or you. It is me and you, me as part of we. I (CCC) like to conclude my meditation practice with the following statement.

> May I be in self-care care.
> May my self-care serve the self-care of others.
> May all beings know and practice self-care.

TIR PRACTICE: CREATING AND MAINTAINING A MANAGEABLE TEACHING SCHEDULE

One of the greatest impediments to mindful self-care is working too much. Sustainability as a yoga teacher requires rest in equal measure to your work. A full-time yoga teacher teaches about 15–20 classes a week, equating to a 40-hour week schedule. General guidance suggests you should not teach more than three classes in one day and have at least one day off a week. As a part-time teacher, it is important to realistically consider your other responsibilities (e.g., childcare, work) as you build your schedule. It may be helpful to offset a weekly yoga class with a training that you offer every six months or yearly that will help you with income. Some teachers also augment with recorded online offerings.

To build your weekly schedule, use the following steps:

1. Look over your practice plan, including your yoga and mindful self-care practices, and add your yoga and mindful self-care practice time into your weekly schedule as a non-negotiable.
2. Write in your other non-negotiables such as childcare and necessary household tasks. If you are a part-time yoga teacher, add in your full-time work responsibilities (e.g., caring for children, work, etc.).
3. Now build in your teaching schedule. No more than three classes a day and at least one day off a week. If you are working full-time and honoring satya (truth) and ahimsa (non-harming), how many classes can you teach and still embody wellbeing? Typically, this is one or two per week maximum.

Re-evaluate your schedule every three months for feasibility. Review the burnout questions and see if your answers have shifted.

TIR PRACTICE: ONGOING PROFESSIONAL DEVELOPMENT AND SUPERVISION

Your 200-hour (and 300- and 500-hour) training is just the beginning of your development as a yoga teacher, not the end. Continuing education is key to your continued growth as a teacher. You are never too old or too experienced to not benefit from continuing education. I (CCC) am writing this book having just returned from a training, where I was a participant, not a leader. Taking the time to situate yourself as a learner, like you are now, will help you be an effective and wise yoga teacher. Yoga Alliance, Yoga International, and many other yoga schools have a host of continuing education opportunities.

At an even deeper level, it is important to get the support and supervision you need. Both writers of this book have teachers and mentors we go to for guidance and support, to untangle philosophies that feel convoluted in the face of today's concerns, and to troubleshoot difficult relationships and challenges. Supervision facilitates competence. A yoga teacher should not wait until they need support. Support should be built into the weekly/monthly schedule as part of professional practice. This supervision/mentorship should be proactive, planned, purposeful, goal-oriented interactions that allow for support and feedback which ultimately facilitate personal growth and growth as a yoga teacher. There are many online resources for this type of supervision; for example:

- Francesca Cervero at www.francescacervero.com
- Kristine Weber, MA, C-IAYT at www.subtleyoga.com
- Joanne Spence, MA, C-IAYT at www.joannespence.com
- Ann Swanson, MS, C-IAYT at www.annswansonwellness.com
- Amy Wheeler, PhD, C-IAYT at https://amywheeler.com

TIR PRACTICE: KNOWING AND REMEMBERING YOUR WHY

Most of us were moved to teach because we believe yoga can be transformational. It is often connected to a personal yoga experience. This is true for both writers of this book. Yoga changed our lives. I (CCC) have felt a longing to share what I know so others don't suffer the way I did before these powerful tools helped me to manage my stressors and challenges, and to love and partner with my body again. Take a moment and close your eyes. Reflect on when you decided you wanted to be a yoga teacher. What was your reasoning? Take a few minutes just breathing and remembering.

MINDFUL SELF-CARE AS A TRAUMA-INFORMED AND RESPONSIVE PRACTICE

Focus on what you feel in your body, the areas around your heart, and your breath. When you are ready, answer the journal prompt below.

> **Journal Prompt.** When did you decide you wanted to be a yoga teacher? Do you remember the moment? Do you remember the reasons why? Do you recall the sensations and feelings in your body? Write them down—when you knew, your reasons why, and how this felt in your body. Last, how does it feel now to remember?

To support your practice, create reminders of your self-care plan and your *why* that you will see regularly. I (CCC) have a mantra on one of my bracelets, notes in my journal, and quotes and reminders in my yoga notebook where I plan my classes. These external reminders can help us remember our *why* on those difficult and long days that can lead us to forget.

Know When You are Impaired, Take a Break, and Get Help

Go back to the questions at the top of the chapter. If you answered yes to some or more of those questions, you may need to take a break and secure mental health support. Explain to your studio or organization that you need to scale back on teaching or take a mental health leave. Take a month or two, maybe more, to get to where you need to be to feel okay and excited about teaching yoga again. As a psychologist and a social worker, the authors of this book strongly believe in the supportive possibility of mental health counseling. There are many effective treatments for anxiety, depression, PTSD, addictions, and other mental health disorders. There is no need to suffer quietly and struggle to get through each day. Last, if at any point you are feeling depressed or suicidal, you must seek help immediately. Dial 988 if you are in the United States to reach the suicide and crisis hotline (most countries have a national number), call a local crisis hotline, or tell someone you love and trust to actively support you and your feelings.

TEACHER TRAINING DISCUSSION QUESTIONS

1. What are the key signs of burnout and compassion fatigue?

2. In what ways could a yoga teacher suffering from burnout be harmful to their yoga students? What is at risk here?
3. What is the scope of practice for a yoga teacher?
4. What types of activities are outside of the yoga teacher's scope of practice?
5. What referrals (business cards, numbers) would be helpful to have in your yoga teaching bag?
6. Why is a personal practice important to your yoga teaching?
7. What is the role of self-care in your professional development and yoga teaching?
8. In what ways are self-care and collective care connected?
9. What factors should you consider when deciding how often you should teach classes each week?

PART II

RESEARCH AND THEORY

Embodiment, Polyvagal Theory, and Sensations

CHAPTER 5

Positive Embodiment, Interoception, and Self-Regulation

yogaå citta-vëtti-nirodhaï

Yoga Sutra I:29

Thence come the awakening of interior consciousness [the true self], and the removal of barriers.

Charles Johnston (1912)

Many yoga teachers and researchers would agree that yoga is an embodied practice and can support positive embodiment. This chapter will review a model of embodiment and define what it means to be positively embodied. The concepts of exteroception, interoception, and neuroception will be introduced along with the concepts of connection and protection as they relate to your nervous system.

Positive Embodiment

The terms *embodied* and *embodiment* are used to describe the felt experience of being human (Cook-Cottone, 2020). We are all embodied to some degree or other, on some spectrum of being positively or dysfunctionally embodied. Embodiment is how we live in, from, through, and with our bodies (Cook-Cottone, 2020). It exists only in the here and now. It includes each of the dimensions of self—your body, feelings, and thoughts—as well as the external aspects of self—your relationships, community, and culture (see Figure 5.1). When you are positively embodied, you have access to voice, choice, and agency.

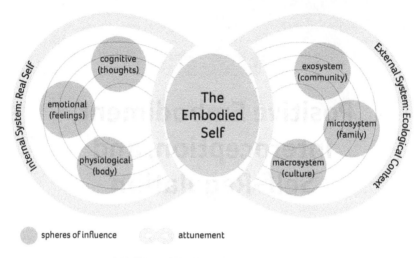

FIGURE 5.1 THE EMBODIED SELF MODEL
(Adapted from Cook-Cottone, 2020)

Positive embodiment requires mindful awareness and intentional action. When a person is positively embodied, they are mindfully aware of all aspects of self, both internally (body, feelings, and thoughts) and externally (family, community, and culture). They connect to all of the aspects of self and use the information accessible through mindful awareness to make choices about how they might *be with* and *work with* in the present, here and now.

A positively embodied person actively practices creating, managing, and supporting attunement among each aspect of self while managing the challenges and experiences of the world around them (see Figure 5.1). A positively embodied person takes care of their body, responding to its needs and wants, giving it time for nourishment and rest, and for challenges and hard work. If you are a positively embodied person, you are attuned to your emotional experiences and can be with and work with your current feelings. You are able to engage in effective thoughts aligning with your psychological emotional experiences *and* facilitate attunement and effective functioning when interacting with others out in the world. Who you are out in the world represents your inner experience. That is, you do not dismiss your internal experience of self when you interface with others. Your interactions with others support your internal wellbeing and pursuit of meaning and purpose in life.

Cook-Cottone defines it this way:

POSITIVE EMBODIMENT, INTEROCEPTION, AND SELF-REGULATION

> *Embodiment* is a way of being, in which being is understood as residing in, and manifesting from, the body as one experiences the internal (i.e., physiological, emotional, cognitive), external (i.e., interpersonal, social, cultural), and existential dimension of life. (2000, p. 1)

Yoga is in essence the experience of positive embodiment in which we abide in our true nature (Sutra 1.2; Ranganathan, 2008). "Yoga, thus, aims at bringing under the control of the person their immediate and proximate environment (the mind and body of the yogi) so that it mirrors the nature of the true self" (Sutra 4.22; Ranganathan, 2008, p. 75).

As we know from our yoga texts, embodiment can shift and change. You can be positively embodied, embodied in a dysfunctional way (binging and purging within the context of an eating disorder), or experience disembodiment or uncanniness (dissociation with trauma). Even when you experience positive embodiment, there will be times when you are internally or externally conflicted, and attunement can be difficult to maintain. For example, your colleague does not show up for the yoga class just after your class. You realize you will now be teaching yoga for three hours straight. You have not been able to eat anything substantial. You feel weak, tired, and emotional. You are not able to attune to your body's needs as you serve the studio and support your friend (who you are either mad at or worried about). You might feel yourself forcing a smile when you tell the studio manager, "Okay, fine, no problem. I can do it." You know you have just lied because it is not fine and you are not okay. The dilemma has pushed you out of your truth (satya). You love to teach yoga from a connected and nourished state of embodiment, yet you find yourself teaching light-headed and hungry, conflicted about your friend, and frustrated with the studio owner. You are not positively embodied.

> **Journal Prompt.** Write about a time when you felt like your internal and external aspects of self were in conflict and you did not take care of yourself. Consider your physiological self (your body), feelings, and thoughts as well as your relationships, community, and perhaps larger culture. What did it feel like? What did you do? If you had the chance to choose differently, how might you have better supported your own positive embodiment?

Trauma is a disintegrating force. It disrupts attuned embodiment and disarms many central aspects of self—thinking, feeling, and being with others. Within many trauma contexts, there is no amount of thinking that can fix things. *The body reacts.* The response is what is called *subcortical*, occurring within the areas beneath the thinking part of the brain. The body's resources are instantaneously allocated protective responses. Emotions, outside of panic and fear, can arrive after the experience or not at all. Trauma can also be an isolating experience. The person experiencing trauma is often separated from anyone who can help or soothe them. As a result, healing and recovery involve reintegrating the experience of self, back into its positively embodied, attuned, and effective self. To do this, a traumatized person needs to understand their nervous system and be able to access loving-kindness with time and practice. As a yoga teacher, your awareness of the effects of trauma and the healing forces of yoga can facilitate a supportive and integrative yoga experience for your students.

> **TIR PRINCIPLE: THE ISSUES ARE IN OUR TISSUES**
> Trauma memories can be stored in the body as nonverbal, physical sensations in muscles and movement, breath patterns, heart rate, feeling-sensations, and action urges.

Listening to Your Body: Interoception, Exteroception, and Neuroception

Living your life from a truly embodied experience requires practice noticing and listening to your body. Your body speaks to you in three main ways: interoception, exteroception, and neuroception.

Interoception, or inside listening, is the process of noticing and listening to sensations inside of your body (Cook-Cottone, 2023; Kube *et al.*, 2020). By listening to the messages coming from inside your body, you will know when you are too hot or too cold, hungry or full, thirsty, need to go to the bathroom, or when your muscles are tired and you need to take a rest. Your interoception is the central way to be responsive to your body's needs. It is one of the main sources of information helping us self-regulate, bringing our bodies to balance (Cook-Cottone, 2023). Interoception can be challenging for those who have experienced trauma. Many people who have experienced trauma describe difficulty turning inward and feeling internal sensations (Cook-Cottone, 2023; Kube *et al.*, 2020). In some cases, they feel

POSITIVE EMBODIMENT, INTEROCEPTION, AND SELF-REGULATION

dissociated from their bodies, feeling nothing at all. In other cases, turning inward can be triggering and overwhelming (Kube *et al.*, 2020). The oft-cited quote "The issues are in our tissues" speaks so clearly to the phenomenon of trauma memories living in our bodies as sensations, muscular tension and movements, breath patterns, heart rates associated with arousal and fear, feeling-sensations reminiscent of the trauma, and action urges, or the urge to do something (Cook-Cottone, 2023).

Exteroception is the process of noticing and listening to the information coming from the world outside of your body (Cook-Cottone, 2023). Your five senses—sight, smell, hearing, touch, and taste—give you information about your environment. Exteroception is a here-and-now process (Cook-Cottone, 2023). Being positively embodied means your communication channels are open, receptive, and responsive through interoception and exteroception.

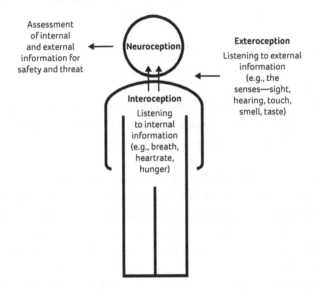

FIGURE 5.2 INTEROCEPTION, EXTEROCEPTION, AND NEUROCEPTION
(Informed by Cook-Cottone, 2023; Kube et al., 2020; Porges, 2021)

Neuroception, a term coined by Stephen Porges, creator of the polyvagal theory (PVT), is the process through which your nervous system assesses safety and threat (Porges, 2017, 2021). It is your body's way of serving as a protector, keeping you safe. Neuroception occurs without conscious awareness. Linked to your body's survival system, it is an automatic process integrating your interoceptive and exteroceptive information. For example, you may be walking to your car in a parking lot, unaware of your neuroceptive process. Suddenly, you notice a gut feeling that something is off (interoception) and you catch unexpected movement in your periphery accompanied by a shuffling sound (exteroception). There is an immediate assessment your body makes related to your safety. Detecting threat or danger, you might freeze (automatically immobilize), move quickly to your car (mobilize), or reflexively orient your awareness toward the area of the visual and auditory stimuli and further assess your safety (orient).

> **TIR PRINCIPLE: NEUROCEPTION**
> Neuroception is the nervous system's automatic process of evaluating safety and threat without requiring awareness.

According to Cook-Cottone (2023), there are two general ways trauma can affect interoception, exteroception, and neuroception:

- **Increased sensitivity:** interoceptive and exteroceptive systems are sensitized to respond to internal and external cues signaling risk or threat *when there is none*.
- **Decreased sensitivity:** interoceptive and exteroceptive systems fail to detect cues that *should* signal risk or threat due to system fatigue, numbness, disconnection, and dissection.

> To illustrate, Kara (she/her) spent months trying to meditate at a park. She had a history of trauma and felt that meditation would help her focus and relax. She would place her towel down, settle herself, take out her meditation beads (also known as mala beads), and close her eyes. Each time, she was unsettled and distracted, and ultimately decided this was an indication of her terrible meditation skills. Then, one day as she returned to her spot to try again, she paused to look around. She noticed a man standing alone. She saw a police car in a parking lot nearby. She overheard a couple arguing. While reflecting on her own experiences growing up in an unsafe home, she realized that her body was telling her there was *potential danger* all around. What she originally thought was her incapability to meditate was her body staying alert and attempting to assess safety. Her history had sensitized her to be alert. Her body was doing its best to secure safety as she sat trying to override it and force a meditation with her eyes closed. From that point forward, she began choosing her meditation spots more carefully and taking a few moments before closing her eyes to scan the area for any potential dangers or triggers. Once she thoughtfully acknowledged her surroundings

(e.g., man waiting for a bus, police car in the parking lot, proximity to people arguing or talking loudly), her body could settle, and she was able to meditate.

> **TIR PRINCIPLE:** ORIENTING FOR SAFETY
> Take a moment before practice to orient for safety.

Orienting for Safety Prior to Practice

This practice can help you (and your students) honor the safety-orienting drives in your body. By taking a moment to orient yourself to your surroundings, you offer the safety-seeking aspects of self to do their job. Note, some people find this very regulating and even calming, and some do not. Trauma-informed and responsive (TIR) techniques are not intended to make everyone feel better in the same way.

Human nervous systems are diverse and have had extraordinarily different experiences and capacities. The goal of TIR techniques is to help students develop tools that work with their nervous systems creating a feeling of self-regulation and attunement with their inner and outer experiences of self (Cook-Cottone, 2015, 2023).

TIR PRACTICE: ORIENTING FOR SAFETY

Select a place to sit comfortably for a short meditation. Before you sit, take a moment to consider the place you have chosen in context. Where is it? Is it a room in a house, near the back of the house? Is it a bench in a park with pathways in front and behind? Intentionally select a location to meditate where you have structure and support behind you. If you are in a room, can you sit with your back to a solid wall (no window or doors)? If you are in a park or outside location, can you find a tree or other structure to support your back? Arrange your materials so you feel well supported (e.g., meditation cushion/bench, blanket, mala beads).

As you sit, begin to use your exteroceptive skills—look, listen, feel. Scan your environment again. Make a note of doorways, pathways, and other access points. You might say to yourself, "I see the door; the door is closed" or "I see people passing 30 feet or so away along the beach." Take time to look to each side, behind you, above you, and on the ground around you. As you do, make a mental note.

Engage your ears. What do you hear coming from each side, above and around you? Do you hear the wind? People chatting? Birds? A dog barking in the distance? You might say to yourself, "I hear the wind and the birds" or "I hear the people talking on the beach."

Pause and breathe. After a few breaths, notice what you feel. Begin from the ground and work your way up. Perhaps you feel a breeze on your skin or through the gentle movement of your hair. You might notice heat radiating from a candle. How does it feel to be in the space or place you are in? Pause and notice.

Bring your awareness to your breath. Meditate here, with a focus on the breath for 3–5 minutes. Allow yourself to pause and scan the environment—sight, sound, and feeling—as you need to. When you do this, consider saying to yourself, "I am orienting for safety." And turn back to your breath. You can close your meditation by honoring your body's efforts to keep you safe. Place your hands on your heart, soften your eyes, and say to yourself, "I honor my body's efforts to keep me safe."

Journal Prompt. What did you notice? How did your body respond to taking a moment to orient for safety before focusing on breath? What did it feel like to honor your body's efforts to keep you safe?

Competing Drives: Connection and Protection

Each day, using your inner awareness (interoception) and awareness of sensations responding to your environment (exteroception), your nervous system is working to ensure your safety. When feeling safe, it is much easier to notice, feel, desire, and engage in connection with others (Cook-Cottone, 2023; Dana, 2020; Porges, 2021). It is easier to feel regulated. Love is the emotion aligned with feelings of connection to ourselves, others, and the world. When feeling threatened or unsafe, the default is defensiveness, withdrawal, agitation, aggression, resistance, and protection. Fear is the emotion aligned with our need to protect ourselves from the parts of ourselves, others, and the world that scare us. As Deb Dana (2020) explains, humans are faced with the ongoing dilemma of balancing our need to survive with our longing for and need to connect with each other. In essence, human beings are constantly balancing two core drives: love and fear.

POSITIVE EMBODIMENT, INTEROCEPTION, AND SELF-REGULATION

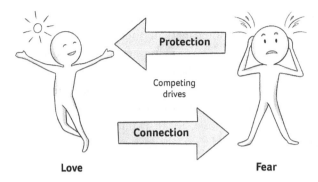

FIGURE 5.3 COMPETING DRIVES: CONNECTION AND PROTECTION
(Informed by Cook-Cottone, 2023; Dana, 2020)

Connection

In 1998, Porges described the social engagement system and referred to the process of that system as love (a bold move in research circles). The social engagement system is how we connect, and when we are most deeply connected, we call this love. Love is the driving force behind our relationship with ourselves, others, and the world. In yoga, we refer to this as loving-kindness (Sutra 1.33; Cook-Cottone, 2015; Ranganathan, 2008).

It is easier to be positively embodied when you are in connection mode. You more readily and openly learn new things, play, and get to know and be with others. Connection is a very important drive for human beings. It supports our relationships and the construction and maintenance of families and communities. When we are born, we are completely vulnerable and depend on other humans to care for us, feed us, and protect us. Without other humans, it is impossible for infants to survive. This means, at the most fundamental levels, we need each other. Human beings thrive because we are able to work in groups. Historically, human beings have accomplished incredible tasks because of our ability to work together. You can see this in architecture, hospital systems, schools and educational systems, and even our yoga communities. When you are in connection mode your number on the self-regulation scale is somewhere between 1 and 6.

Protection

Our protective mode is important to our survival. In this mode, our nervous system is oriented toward potential threats, and its main functions are safety and survival (Dana, 2020). The primary feeling associated with protection mode is fear. Fear is one of the main disruptors of positive embodiment and increases nervous system dysregulation. In the yoga sutras, fear represents our attachment, or clinging to bodily security, our need for physical and emotional safety (Sutra 2.3; Ranganathan, 2008). There are many things and experiences that frighten humans—flying, heights, aggressive or frightened animals, and lightning storms. The most complicated, however, is the fear associated with our interactions with other humans. As much as we need other humans, the most likely cause of harm to any human is, in fact, another human (Cook-Cottone, 2023). Trauma can sensitize a person to be primarily oriented toward the protective mode.

TEACHER TRAINING DISCUSSION QUESTIONS

1. What does the term *positive embodiment* mean to you?
2. How does yoga help you to be more positively embodied?
3. Explain how and why trauma can be a disintegrating force.
4. Describe the difference between exteroception, interoception, and neuroception.
5. How might you apply the self-regulation scale to how you relate to yourself and your yoga students?
6. Name and explain the competing drives of the nervous system.

CHAPTER 6

Polyvagal Theory, Window of Tolerance, and Co-Regulation

vitarka-vicârânandâsmitâ-rûpânugamât samprajõâtaï

Yoga Sutra 1:17

Meditation with an object follows these stages: first, exterior examining, then interior judicial action, then joy, then realization of individual being.

Charles Johnston (1912)

In order for you to be effectively trauma-informed and responsive (TIR), you will need a solid understanding of three concepts: the polyvagal theory (PVT), the window of tolerance, and co-regulation. The polyvagal theory, introduced by Stephen Porges (2021), will help you understand how our nervous system works on a day-to-day basis to gear up for the day, manage challenges, stay alert and engaged, and wind down and relax. It will also help you understand how trauma and extreme stress are managed by the nervous system. The window of tolerance is a concept introduced by Daniel Siegel (2010) and Pat Ogden (2021). This concept is very helpful when combined with the PVT, explaining how and why the nervous system shifts from day-to-day functions to stress- and trauma-related reactions. Last, the co-regulation concept explains the power and impact of your way of being with and connecting to your body within the yoga session. This chapter will detail each concept and help you begin applying these concepts to your understanding of your own nervous systems and the nervous systems of your yoga students.

> **TIR PRINCIPLE:** POLYVAGAL THEORY
> Take time to know, understand, and apply the polyvagal theory to yourself and your students.

The Nervous System, Trauma, and Yoga: The Science and Theory

Perhaps one of the most groundbreaking theories to enter the fields of embodiment, yoga, and trauma work is the polyvagal theory (PVT) by Stephen Porges (2021) which explains what happens within the body and mind across the comfort and growth zones (detailed below) and outside the window of tolerance. The PVT provides a theoretical foundation for brain-body science and practices such as yoga. Porges described his excitement regarding the use of the PVT in mental and physical health treatment models, saying, "This strategy would focus on recruiting the nervous system of the client or patients as a collaboration on a shared journey toward wellness" (2021, p. xv). Porges' theory was groundbreaking with emphasis on the bi-directional communication system between the brain and body: "eighty percent of the fibers in the vagus nerve arise from the body and travel towards the brain and the other twenty percent originate from the brain to the body" (Spence, 2021, p. 40). This means the body has a huge influence over the brain, more so than the other way around. Bi-directional communication of the vagus nerve provides an explanation as to why yoga poses with connection to one's breath provide direct access to the nervous system. As Porges (2017) emphasizes, controlling the breath provides immediate access to the autonomic nervous system, creating the potential for state change. In Chapters 15, 16, and 17, you will learn more about which yoga postures and breathing practices can create specific state changes to the autonomic nervous system.

As taught during the physiology and anatomy sections of yoga teacher training, there are two main components of the nervous system: the central nervous system (brain and spinal cord) and the peripheral nervous system (see Figure 6.1). The peripheral nervous system branches into the somatic nervous system and the autonomic nervous system. The PVT focuses on the functions of the autonomic nervous system (ANS).

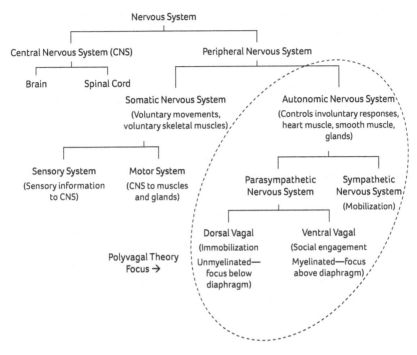

FIGURE 6.1 THE NERVOUS SYSTEM AND THE POLYVAGAL THEORY FOCUS

The ANS works automatically, often below awareness (Cook-Cottone, 2023). It keeps your heart beating and lungs breathing in attunement with internal and external needs, demands, and challenges. It is in charge of responding to safety and danger. The functions of the ANS can be deeply impacted by trauma, making it more sensitive and reactive (Cook-Cottone, 2023). Your autonomic nervous system is made of two nervous systems: *sympathetic* and *parasympathetic* (see Figure 6.1).

Sympathetic nervous system. The sympathetic nervous system is your mobilizer—the get-going part of your nervous system. It helps you in connection and protection modes. It supports, responds to, and regulates blood circulation, heart rhythm, body temperature, blood flow to large muscle groups, sweating, vigilance, and posture changes. When necessary, it can decrease blood flow to parts of the body like your gastrointestinal systems and skin (your fingers might get cold). Overall, it helps you get alert and moving while also gearing you up in matters of passion and play. When you are in danger or feel threatened, the sympathetic nervous system mobilizes you to a state of fight or flight. It works with the parasympathetic nervous system during the freeze response, creating an elevated sense of alertness preparing you for fight or flight.

Key takeaways:

- The sympathetic nervous system helps you get going (mobilize).
- When you are in danger, it mobilizes you into fight or flight states.
- When you are in danger, it supports alertness and preparation in the freeze state.

Parasympathetic nervous system. According to the PVT, the parasympathetic nervous system is your calm-down, slow-down system, or immobilizer. The PVT posits that this system helps you connect to others and in keeping you safe. The PVT gets its name from the vagus nerve. More than a single nerve, it is really a group of neural pathways with nerve fibers that wander, or extend, throughout the core of your body facilitating communication between your body and brain. PVT holds that the vagus nerve divides into two circuits: the ventral vagal complex (VVC) and the dorsal vagal complex (DVC).

Key takeaways:

- The parasympathetic nervous system calms and slows you down (immobilize), helps you connect to yourself and others, and plays a role in maintaining safety.
- It is made of two circuits or complexes—the ventral vagal complex (VVC) and the dorsal vagal complex (DVC).

The PVT explains how the sympathetic and parasympathetic (VVC and DVC) nervous systems work together to help you maintain day-to-day functioning, gear up for challenges and safety concerns, focus at work or school, have fun with friends, connect to loved ones, and relax and restore when you need to (Dana, 2020; Porges, 2021; Spence, 2021; see Figure 6.1). Specific circumstances determine when each system takes over and runs the show.

The ventral vagal complex. The VVC is the myelinated (insulated) branch of the vagus nerve, allowing it to send information quickly. The VVC is associated with the parts of your body above the diaphragm. When the VVC is active, your nervous system works in ways supporting health, growth, restoration, and connectedness to self and others (Cook-Cottone, 2023; Dana, 2020; Porges, 2021). As Porges (2021) explains, the VVC evolved when mammals diverged from our reptile ancestors, developing a face–heart connection linking the heart, lungs, throat and vocal cords, inner ear, and facial muscles around our mouth and eyes (Cook-Cottone, 2023; Dana, 2020; Porges, 2021). The VVC is often referred to as the *social engagement system* because it helps you connect and communicate with others through its control of the muscles in your face (including how you show emotions), the pitch and tone of your voice, the nature of the look in your eyes, and the subtle tilts of your head (Cook-Cottone, 2023; Spence, 2021). Researchers and mental health professionals are very interested in the VVC; when it runs the show, you are your most healthy, happy, flexible, and adaptive. As a yoga teacher, you want to actively cultivate your VVC state when preparing to teach. When the VVC is active, it is easier to make choices supporting your wellbeing, receive and offer support to others, and assess safety and threat more accurately (Cook-Cottone, 2023). It is important to note the VVC is *not* active during fight or flight or when a person is reacting to trauma or a trauma memory.

Key takeaways:

- Activation of the ventral vagal complex (VVC) helps you connect to yourself and others.
- Day to day, when the VVC is active, you are healthier, happier, more flexible, adaptive, and able to make healthier choices.
- Under duress, the VVC can become inactive.

The dorsal vagal complex. The DVC is the immobilization, or *calm-down, slow-down,* complex. It consists of the unmyelinated (non-insulated) branch, making it slower (Porges, 2021). It connects to the organs that are below your diaphragm and sends a smaller number of nerve fibers to your heart (Cook-Cottone, 2023; Porges, 2021). Generally, during day-to-day experiences, the DVC can be thought of as a software program that runs in the background: regulating digestion, supporting rest, and facilitating healing. During extremely stressful or potentially dangerous situations, the DVC works with the sympathetic nervous system in activating a freeze response. Movement, heart rate, and breathing are reduced while the sympathetic nervous system supports alertness and preparations for action. Under extreme stress or overwhelming threat, the DVC activates the shutdown response, experienced as numbness, dissociation, fainting, or collapse (Cook-Cottone, 2023; Dana, 2020; Porges, 2021; Spence, 2021). This shutdown response has been referred to as a *dorsal dive* in other mammals; it is also called death feigning (e.g., possums).

Key takeaways:

- Day to day, the dorsal vagal complex (DVC) runs in the background, helping your body rest, digest, and heal.
- Under extreme duress, the DVC activates the freeze and shutdown responses.

Table 6.1 brings all of this science and theory together for you. You can see both connection and protection modes, the associated states of embodiment, and the body experiences present as parasympathetic and sympathetic nervous systems work together to keep you connected and protected. On the right is a column that indicates the associated number of the self-regulation scale.

Table 6.1 States of Embodiment and the Active Polyvagal Pathways

State of Embodiment	What It Feels Like	Autonomic Nervous System Actions	SRS*	Mode
Connection States				
Rest, restoration, and recovery	Safe and relaxed	Ventral vagal connection and intentional dorsal vagal (PNS) immobilization	1	C O N N E C T I O N
			2	
Alert engagement	Safe	Ventral vagal (PNS) connection and intentional, mild sympathetic mobilization	3	
Challenge and growth	Safe and Activated	Ventral vagal (PNS) connection and intentional, moderate sympathetic mobilization	4	
			5	
			6	

Protection States

			SRS*	
Fight or flight	Unsafe and threatened	Strong sympathetic mobilization	7	
			8	P R O T E C T I O N
Freeze	Unsafe and threatened	Dorsal vagal (PNS) immobilization and sympathetic alertness and preparation		
			9	
Shutdown	Overloaded and overwhelmed	Strong dorsal vagal (PNS) immobilization spike in response to incapacitated sympathetic response	10	

(*SRS = self-regulation scale)
(*Informed by Cook-Cottone, 2020, 2023; Dana, 2020; Porges, 2021*)

Exploring Your Connection and Protection States

The PVT is complicated and can be difficult to get your head around. Figure 6.2 offers another way of looking at it. The top of the vertical axis represents the activation of the sympathetic nervous system (the get-going part of your nervous system). The bottom of the vertical axis represents DVC activation (your calm-down, slow-down complex). The horizontal axis represents VVC activation (right) and deactivation (left).

When you are feeling safe, you can experience both activation and deactivation of your sympathetic nervous system (Cook-Cottone, 2023). This can feel like getting excited and settling down, all while feeling connected to yourself and others (the upper right side of the figure). This is called *mobilization without fear*. You can also feel calm and connected while being relaxed, resting, and restoring (the lower right side of the figure). This is called *immobilization without fear*.

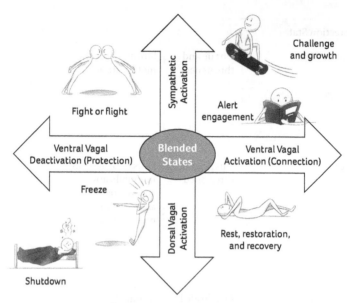

FIGURE 6.2 POLYVAGAL BLENDED STATES
(Informed by Cook-Cottone, 2023; Dana, 2020; Porges, 2021)

> **TIR PRINCIPLE: CONNECTION AND PROTECTION**
> Those who have been through trauma are sensitized toward protection over connection.

After experiencing trauma, a person's nervous system can become sensitized and may react more strongly to stressors and triggers (Cook-Cottone, 2023). As a result, the body is likely to shift into a protection state more often than it needs (the left side of Figure 6.2), and more than perhaps the person would like. Accordingly, a person who has been through trauma spends more time on the left side of Figure 6.2. The top left represents the fight or flight response, which is *mobilization in reaction to fear* (Cook-Cottone, 2023). The bottom left presents freeze and shutdown, which is *immobilization in reaction to fear*. Most of us, whether or not we have been through trauma, have experienced each of these states.

In order to help you internalize what each of these states feels like in your own body (which will help you better recognize them in your students' bodies), below we will guide you through an exploration of each. As you read, you will notice the states of the body and nervous system are associated with particular feelings and thoughts. Body states affect feelings and thoughts, just as feelings and thoughts affect body states. In fact, a person's thoughts, feelings, and body states are key access points for self-regulation (see Figure 6.3).

Body states are the most overlooked, by traditional psychological approaches to wellbeing, and perhaps the most powerful access point. Yoga approaches work directly with body states and this, in part, is why they are so self-regulating and healing and why so many psychologists and mental health professionals have begun to integrate yoga techniques into their practice (Spence, 2021).

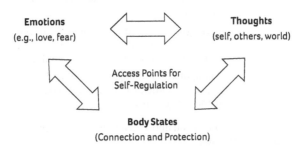

FIGURE 6.3 ACCESS POINTS FOR SELF-REGULATION

TIR PRACTICE: SEEING BODY (PVT) STATES IN THE YOGA SESSION

Table 6.2 is an activity to help you connect the PVT states to your yoga teaching. This table builds on the previous table detailing the PVT above. Read through each state. Consider how the three access points for self-regulation (body states, emotions, and thoughts) affect each other in each state. Next, in the space provided, write what you might notice if one of your yoga students was in that state. Describe what you might notice about how they are holding their body, their facial expression, breath rate, sweating, movements, and other behaviors. Being able to identify body states in your students is a central foundational skill in TIR yoga teaching and it takes time and practice to develop.

Table 6.2 Understanding the Embodied States

Connection States	
Rest, Restoration, and Recovery 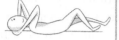	**Body:** The state of rest, restoration, and recovery occurs during deeply relaxing moments as in *Savasana* (lying down pose) at the end of a yoga class (Cook-Cottone, 2023). In this state, your body is likely responding to cues of safety such as the yoga teacher's kind and gentle voice or the accepting and well-supported feeling of the yoga space (Cook-Cottone, 2023). Although this is different for everyone, other experiences eliciting this state can include cuddling, petting a dog or cat, a massage, and a warm bath. The body softens and relaxes, allowing restorative systems to engage. The body can rest, digest, and heal. **Feelings:** You feel safe and connected to yourself and others. Feelings in this state include contentment, peacefulness, warmth, and loving-kindness. **Thoughts:** Your thoughts are soft and restful—"I am at peace," "Other people are kind and loving," or "The world is a good place."

In a yoga class, what signs might you notice that indicate a student is in the rest, restoration, and recovery state?

Alert Engagement 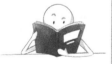	**Body:** When you are in the alert engagement state, you feel integrated and effective. You feel aligned as you sense, feel, and think (Cook-Cottone, 2023). The part of the brain that thinks and conceptualizes (neocortex) and the part of the brain that processes emotions (limbic system) easily communicate with each other (Cook-Cottone, 2023). **Feelings:** You feel safe and connected to yourself and others. It feels manageable to experience your emotions and learn from them, be creative, and feel a sense of open-heartedness. **Thoughts:** Your thoughts include a sense of empowerment and possibility—"I can do this," "I am excited to work with others," and "If we work together, we can solve larger problems in this world."

In a yoga class, what signs might you notice that indicate a student is in the alert engagement state?

POLYVAGAL THEORY, WINDOW OF TOLERANCE, AND CO-REGULATION

Challenge and Growth 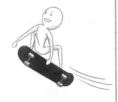	**Body:** In this state, you are engaged, connected, and challenged as you learn something new, play a sport, or engage in something difficult (Cook-Cottone, 2023). Your muscles and your nervous system are activated. **Feelings:** You feel the thrill of the challenge. Feelings are generally positive such as happy and excited. There can also be times when you feel challenge, frustration, and irritability. **Thoughts:** Thoughts acknowledge the challenge as well as the possibility—"This is difficult. I am focused and I can try," "I am going to figure out how I can work with this person," and "The world is a challenging and exciting place."

In a yoga class, what signs might you notice that indicate a student is in the challenge and growth state?

Protection States	
Fight or Flight 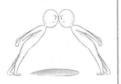	**Body:** The body moves into a highly efficient state of fight or flight. The digestive and immune systems are suppressed. The body prioritizes large gross motor muscles that support running and fighting. The heart beats fast, breath rate increases (or breath holding), jaws clench, eyes harden, and you become very aware of your environment. The thinking part of the brain (frontal orbital cortex) is inhibited and the feeling or reactive part of the brain (the limbic system) is activated (Cook-Cottone, 2023). Some people describe this as an amygdala hijack. **Feelings:** The feelings often present in this state include fear, agitation, annoyance, impatience, anger, hate, rage, terror, and threat. Afterwards, when the thinking brain is back online, we are left with regret, embarrassment, and sometimes shame. **Thinking:** Thoughts include "I am not safe," "People are not safe," and "The world is not a safe place." There may also be absence of thoughts or thoughts racing.

In a yoga class, what signs might you notice that indicate a student is in the fight or flight state?

cont.

TRAUMA-INFORMED AND TRAUMA-RESPONSIVE YOGA TEACHING

Protection States	
Freeze 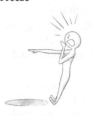	**Body:** Through neuroception, the brain and body have determined there is no escape and fighting would not ensure survival (Cook-Cottone, 2023). The body is immobilized. The body becomes very still and alert; muscles tense as if in preparation for a fight or an escape. **Feelings:** Feelings can range from feeling nothing (numb) to experiencing extreme fear. **Thoughts:** Like feelings, there can be no thoughts at all or thoughts about lack of safety.

In a yoga class, what signs might you notice that indicate a student is in the freeze state?

Shutdown 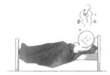	**Body:** Shutdown is sometimes referred to as behavioral collapse (Cook-Cottone, 2023). It can be experienced as an inability to speak or move, fainting, losing consciousness, and/or dissociation (i.e., disconnection from the present moment, awareness, thoughts, memories, the environment, and/or actions). At this extreme end of protection mode, the body is focusing on survival. The body decreases blood flow and oxygen to the large muscle groups, preserving them to send to the brain. **Feelings:** Feelings in this state include feeling nothing, incapacitation, terror, or utter overwhelm. **Thoughts:** In this state, there are often few or no coherent thoughts.

In a yoga class, what signs might you notice that indicate a student is in the shutdown state?

Window of Tolerance, Comfort Zone, and Growth Zone

Now that we have considered the PVT and how the different states might present in a yoga class, let's consider the experience of moving from one state to another. The window of tolerance, comfort zone, and growth zone are three very important TIR yoga teaching concepts/tools. These terms will give you language and tools that will help you identify what you are seeing as you notice and respond to your students and your own levels of activation as you teach.

Window of tolerance. A person's window of tolerance is the range of activation within which you can remain positively embodied, aligned with loving-kindness, and in the connection mode. The term is used by both Pat Ogden (2021), the developer of Sensorimotor Psychotherapy, and Dan Siegel (2010), an expert in interpersonal neurobiology. The window of tolerance is the current level of challenge or stress that you can manage as you get through the day, negotiate challenges, and work on your healing and recovery (see Figure 6.4). It begins with your comfort and growth zones, in which you are solidly in connection mode and able to connect to self and others.

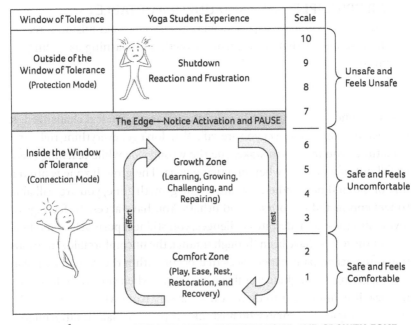

FIGURE 6.4 WINDOW OF TOLERANCE, COMFORT ZONE, AND GROWTH ZONE

Comfort zone. When you are in your comfort zone, you feel a sense of ease. You feel comfortable. You can freely play, rest, restore, and recover here. You have a sense of mastery in your comfort zone. You can connect to yourself and others. Feelings of loving-kindness are easily accessible, and you feel positively embodied. This corresponds to a Self-Regulation Scale Score of 1 or 2 (Cook-Cottone, 2023). Most of us really like being in our comfort zones. It feels safe and good.

> **Journal Prompt.** Take a moment and recall a time when you felt that you were in your comfort zone. Perhaps you were practicing a yoga posture you know well. Describe what it felt like to be in your comfort zone. As you think back, what do you notice in your body? How do you feel emotionally? How would you describe the thoughts that you noticed?

> **TIR PRINCIPLE: SAFE AND UNCOMFORTABLE**
> Individuals who have experienced trauma sometimes misinterpret the discomfort that comes from growth and learning as feeling unsafe.

Growth zone. When you are in your growth zone, you feel challenged. It can feel uncomfortable, yet you are safe. You don't get everything right and sometimes you make a mistake, cue the wrong side while teaching class, or fall out of a posture when practicing yoga. The growth zone is often a mix of old and new. When you are in the growth zone, you are still able to feel connected to yourself and others. You have access to feelings of loving-kindness and, despite challenges, you still feel positively embodied.

For those who have been through trauma, the uncomfortable sensations that often accompany experiences that occur within the growth zone can feel triggering—it might feel as if you are unsafe when you are, in fact, safe. In yoga, it is important to discern what is safe from what is unsafe. The classic example of the man who mistook a rope for a snake is often offered to illustrate yoga sutra 1.8 ("Illusion is the improper comprehension of real objects not based on their true forms"; Ranganathan, 2008, pp. 80–81). As Ranganathan (2008) explains, when we mistake a rope for a snake, we have correctly noticed a characteristic of the object—this is a long, thin, and twisting shape. Our error, however, is in our conclusion that we have observed a snake. In the same way, after experiencing trauma, it can be very easy to experience discomfort as threatening or unsafe. *When we make this error, we are at risk of abandoning our growth zone and withdrawing into our comfort zone where everything feels safe.*

> **Journal Prompt.** Take a moment and recall a time when you felt that you were in your growth zone. Perhaps you were learning something new or you were doing something you know how to do with new people or in a new place. Describe what it felt like to be in your growth zone. As you think back, what do you notice in your body? How do you feel emotionally? How would you describe the thoughts that you noticed?

The cycle of effort and rest. Yoga is the practice of moving in and out of our comfort and growth zones. As you do this, you embody the cycle of rest and effort. We learn to discern between what is safe, comfortable, uncomfortable, and unsafe. We learn the internal signals that inform us it's time to rest and the signals say we are ready for a challenge. This zone corresponds to a Self-Regulation Scale Score of 3, 4, 5, or 6, depending on how activated you might feel. At the lower end, closer to your comfort zone, you will likely feel more confident as you address a challenge (i.e., 3 or 4). At the higher end (i.e., 5 or 6), you might feel yourself getting frustrated, anxious, and on your way to being overwhelmed. These are all signs that you are getting close to the edge of your window of tolerance.

> **TIR PRINCIPLE: GREAT EFFORT AND GREAT REST**
> Sustainability is supported by cycling periods of effort and rest. Effort enhances rest and rest supports effort.

The edge of the window of tolerance. There is a place between your growth zone and outside of your window of tolerance. This is your edge. Perhaps this is one of the most important points of awareness within yourself and with your yoga students. At the edge of the window of tolerance, you and your students will still, potentially, have the awareness and resources to notice your activation level (i.e., Self-Awareness Scale Score of 7). You might notice your heart starting to race and your muscle tension increasing; you might sweat; and your emotions might begin to feel strong and possibly a bit overwhelming. Interestingly, it can become more difficult to notice and be aware as you are increasingly activated. This is why it can be very helpful for you and your yoga students to take a PAUSE before you get to your edge.

TRAUMA-INFORMED AND TRAUMA-RESPONSIVE YOGA TEACHING

> **Journal Prompt.** Take a moment and recall a time when you felt that you were close to the edge of your window of tolerance. What were the signals you noticed? As you think back, what do you notice in your body? How do you feel emotionally? How would you describe the thoughts that you noticed?

Outside of your window of tolerance. When you or your yoga students are outside of the window of tolerance, you enter a reactive and protective state of being. Emotions and behaviors can feel out of control. This can feel like panic, complete overwhelm, or shutdown and collapse. When individuals are outside of their window of tolerance, they can feel disembodied. It can be extremely difficult, if not impossible, to integrate the aspects of self—body, emotions, and thoughts. It is a disintegrating experience. The reactions occurring outside of the window of tolerance do not reflect a person's true intentions or values because the thinking parts of the brain are unable to effectively contribute to decision making. On the Self-Awareness Scale, this zone is scored 8, 9, or 10, depending on level of activation and overwhelm.

> **PRACTICING THE PAUSE**
> Any time, any place, and for any reason, you can always PAUSE. Pause = stop what you are doing, A = assess how you are and what you need, and USE = use your resources.

TIR Yoga Teaching and Co-Regulation

As a TIR yoga teacher, the student is able to experience a range of emotions and activation levels and states, and experiment with being with and working with them. It is this attunement, resonance, and reciprocation that is at the heart of teaching yoga in a trauma-informed and responsive manner. As the yoga teacher, you continuously work on your embodied presence so you can be grounded, aware, and engaged. You work to create a container of safety for and responsiveness to your students. You are self-regulated and are able to keep your social engagement system, your connection mode, activated. Your awareness of the students includes awareness of their body states (physiology), emotions, and thoughts. You are attuned to them. Your cues and guidance reflect your insight into their experience. Through repeated experiences, your students may experience a sensation of safety and trust, facilitating activation of their social engagement, or connection, systems. This enhances their ability to stay connected to self and others as they explore the range of body states, emotions, and thoughts that arise when a person is truly being with and connected to their own body.

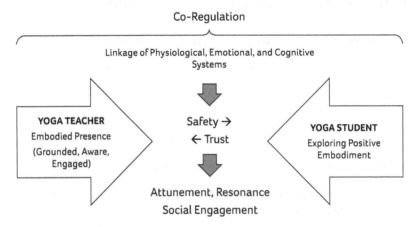

FIGURE 6.5 CO-REGULATION OF YOGA TEACHER AND STUDENT

Ultimately, as TIR yoga teachers, we hope to give students tools to be self-regulated in service of their own needs, wants, and sense of meaning. Through the practice of yoga, students can move through mobility and immobility in a self-directed and empowered manner. Choice—*authentic and real choice*—arises from the ability to be aware inside (interoception) and outside (exteroception), and to make choices based on what is noticed and where one is headed (e.g., "I am working toward a challenging pose," "I seek relaxation," "I am here to strengthen my core and gain mobility," "I am here to learn about the philosophy of yoga"). The reason comes from the students. We, as yoga teachers, facilitate and support their experiences. Their path is a courageous one. Where yoga takes each of us can be a very powerful place indeed.

Arielle Schwartz illustrates the level of self-discovery that is possible through her yoga practice in her book *Therapeutic Yoga for Trauma Recovery*:

> Your postures, breath practices, and meditations help you awaken to the essence of who you really are. You move past your physical armor, emotional tension, and mental activity as you make your way to the very center of your being. (2022, p. 144)

If you really enjoy reading about the PVT, check out the work of Deb Dana (2020) who does a wonderful job of explaining the PVT in an understandable way. Both Stephen Porges' (2021) and Deb Dana's (2020) texts are excellent resources.

TEACHER TRAINING DISCUSSION QUESTIONS

1. Describe what an embodied state is. Give two examples.
2. What are the connection and protection states? Give examples of how these states might present in a yoga student.
3. What are the three access points for self-regulation?
4. Why is polyvagal theory important to you as a yoga teacher?
5. How might the window of tolerance relate to your yoga teaching?
6. Describe the difference between your comfort zone and your growth zone. Give examples of each.
7. How might you use the principle of great effort and great rest in yoga practice and teaching?
8. What is co-regulation?

CHAPTER 7

Sensations—The Basics

draæøë-dëåyayoï saäyogo heya-hetuï

Yoga Sutra II:17

The cause of what is to be warded off [suffering], is the absorption of the Seer [witness] in things seen [what is witnessed].

Charles Johnston (1912)

In this chapter, you will learn about sensations and their key traits. Sensations are central to trauma-informed and responsive (TIR) practices. They are the pathway through which our bodies transmit stimuli to our perceptual systems (e.g., exteroception, interoception, and neuroception).

Stimuli (from inside/outside) → **Sensation** → **Perception** (e.g., extero-, intero-, neuroception)

We all have our own unique bodies, histories, and experiences that affect how we process the world and all of its sensational experiences. Sensations are intricately linked to the practice of yoga and learning to connect to our bodies. To truly know the body, you must be able to listen to its messengers: sensations. Sensations are communications telling us the state of our physiological and emotional aspects of our embodied self. *Trauma can cause a person to be overly sensitive to and/or under-responsive to sensations.*

When a student enters a yoga class, they have entered the world of sensations. As teachers, we guide students to orient toward the sensations related to breath, tensions and relaxation, injuries and pain, open-heartedness, emotional defensiveness, and, sometimes, traumatic and physical memories. Many believe this to be one of the strongest mechanisms of change associated with yoga practice. Through your sensations, yoga is a uniquely powerful way to deeply connect with your body.

> **TIR PRINCIPLE: SENSATIONS ARE COMMUNICATIONS**
> Our bodies communicate the state of our physiological and emotional selves through sensations.

Understanding Sensations: A Conceptual Tool for Embodied Self-Regulation

Sensations are a critical pathway to knowing yourself, others, and the world. To be self-regulated, an individual must develop the capacity to be aware of sensations, their qualities, and their role in self-regulation. Yoga is *sensational*. Each form of yoga practice (i.e., asana, breathwork, meditation) yields an abundance of sensations. When anyone practices yoga, they are practicing *being with* and *working with* sensations of all kinds. Some of these sensations are related to the pose (or practice) and the present moment. Others are related to internal needs, past events, emotions, and state activation. We'll start here with a basic overview of sensations.

Key Traits of Sensations

Embodied self-regulation is about recognizing and being with sensations as they arise and pass. No matter what their origin or function, all sensations share several key traits.

1. Sensations give us information about ourselves, our relationships, and our world.
2. Sensations can be noticed, described, considered, and explored.
3. Sensations can be comfortable, neutral, and uncomfortable.
4. Sensations can be associated with action urges, a desire to do something.
5. Sensations arise and pass.

Trait #1: Sensations give us information about ourselves, our relationships, and our world

TIR yoga teaching integrates consistent cueing, orienting students to their sensations. We will be detailing cueing in a future chapter. Here, we're highlighting the *why* of this practice. Being aware of and listening to sensations helps yoga students make choices. If you do not know what you are feeling and experiencing, it is quite difficult, if not impossible, to be fully self-determined. Consider this question: how would a student know how to safely deepen into a pose, stay, or ease out, if they are not linking this choice to the sensations noticed in the joints involved? When well practiced, this same type of sensation-informed personal decision making can be taken off the mat and into the world. For example, you might get better at noticing feelings in your gut telling you that something is not right. Sensations are central to this type of embodied wisdom (Cook-Cottone, 2023).

Trait #2: Sensations can be noticed, described, considered, and explored
Yoga teachers can help students learn to notice, describe, consider, and explore sensations. When you move toward noticing your sensations and away from reacting to them, you begin to feel more self-regulated. Noticing, rather than reacting, gives you, and your yoga students, the space to make choices. There are many characteristics to notice about sensations. You can notice many qualities within sensations (Cook-Cottone, 2023). These include the fundamental qualities like size, shape, solidity, temperature, color, smell, taste, sound, humidity, weight, sharpness, texture. There are also secondary qualities such as pain level, stability, organization, motion, and intensity (Cook-Cottone, 2023).

> When Sam (they/them) was a beginning yoga student, holding Warrior Pose 1 (*Virabhadrasana 1*) was very challenging, especially in their shoulders and upper arms. They often got reactive and began thinking thoughts like "My arms are weak," "This is uncomfortable," and "I hate this pose." Through many reminders from their teacher and many yoga practices, Sam shifted their relationship with Warrior I. They began to notice the work their shoulders and upper arms were doing, and supported their muscles by adding slow, steady breaths. They thought, "I notice my arms working hard. I will breathe to support them." Sam noticed what it felt like for their muscles to contract, their heart to beat, and breath to move in and out of their body as they worked. When they felt that it was time to release the pose, they did. This was a powerful shift for Sam. They felt a sense of partnership with and ownership over their own body. They did not need to react or judge. Sam could be with and work with exactly what was present.

Trait #3: Sensations can be comfortable, neutral, and uncomfortable
In a wonderful theoretical article, Grabovac *et al.* (2011) describe the Buddhist Psychological Model. This model describes the process of noticing sensations (Grabovac refers to this as a sense impression). As you become aware of each arising sensation, the brain automatically tags it as pleasant, unpleasant, or neutral. This tagging leads us to habitually approach or avoid

the sensations (i.e., attachment and aversion). In their model, this pattern continues automatically for each sensation and each sensation-related thought, leading to what they call mental proliferation, or ruminating.

> To illustrate, Sam is doing Warrior Pose 2 (*Virabhadrasana 2*). They notice the sensation of their deltoids working hard. Their brain tags that sensation as unpleasant. This leads to avoidance and the thought "My arms are weak, and I hate this pose." Thinking those thoughts is unpleasant, which leads to a stronger urge to avoid. They then think, "I am not good at yoga. I should not be here." This is unpleasant and leads to more avoidance. Their body begins to get reactive and defensive. Their muscles tense. Their breath becomes shallow. Their heart rate increases. Their brain tags more unpleasantness. And so it goes.
>
> Once Sam began reacting to the sensations in their shoulders, not being with and exploring these sensations, they got lost in rumination. One thought after another reinforced the negative and reactive cycle taking them far away from the present moment.

Like Sam, we all get stuck on our reactions to sensations and thoughts without experiencing them as they are. In order to stop this automatic and habitual process, we practice being with sensations as they arise and pass. We give ourselves support, ground with our feet, and focus on our breath. We let go of any need to attach or avoid and work to accept the moment exactly as it is. We now have space to make choices connected to what is best for the body and mind in this moment—we are not lost in reactive and ruminative (i.e., compulsive thinking, the same thoughts over and over) patterns. Grabovac and colleagues (2011) refer to this shift as acceptance and attentional regulation.

> **TIR PRINCIPLE: SENSATIONS AND SAFETY**
> There is no universal relationship between safety and sensations that can be applied to all people.

It would be wonderful if sensations could accurately and specifically speak to safety at all times. Unfortunately, they can't. In TIR yoga teaching, we acknowledge that working with unpleasant sensations can be complicated. See Figure 7.1: whether a pose is safe, risky, or unsafe doesn't always align with a certain sensational tone. A person with a trauma history might not feel sensations easily and cannot use sensations to determine if a pose or practice feels safe, risky, or unsafe. Someone who hurt their shoulder six months ago might experience shoulder work as unpleasant and consider some safe poses unsafe because of the unpleasant sensations. Or certain poses really are unsafe and their interpretation of the sensations are 100 percent correct. Someone who is 75 years old might know their body well and choose not to do Camel Pose due to the impact on their knees. A yoga student may have a collagen disorder and, despite being young and strong, experience forward folds and their hips very differently from a person without the disorder.

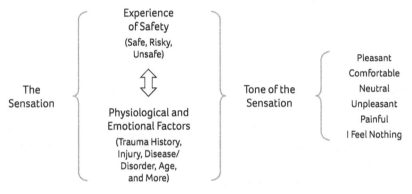

FIGURE 7.1 FACTORS AFFECTING THE RELATIONSHIP BETWEEN THE SENSATION AND THE TONE

Recall, it is very easy for someone who has experienced trauma to feel something uncomfortable as unsafe. Their window of tolerance is often small, and it can be difficult to tolerate sensations that others can tolerate easily. As yoga students develop skills for feeling uncomfortable as they grow, their window of tolerance will expand. Each and every student in the yoga class will have a different history and distinct window of tolerance. The choice point (to stay in *Savasana* or go, to work through Warrior II or release the pose) for any given student can be quite different. Critically, the goal of TIR yoga teaching is not to help students go to the depths of every pose, or to hold poses for an increasingly longer period of time. It is not to develop the capacity to endure pain and discomfort. The goal is to support the processes of self-regulation, integration, attunement with the body, befriending the body, and making choices that are deeply connected to the wellbeing of self and others.

Ultimately, there are two competing truths here. First, there is no universal relationship between safety and sensations applicable to all people.

Second, working with discomfort and your reactions to it is critical for your growth and healing.

> **TIR PRINCIPLE:** DISCOMFORT AND GROWTH
> Working with discomfort and reactions to it is critical for growth and healing.

Trait #4: Sensations can be associated with action urges, a desire to do something

Sensations often come with an action urge. An action urge is the desire to do something based on the sensation you are experiencing (Cook-Cottone, 2023). For example, when you are angry, you might feel your hands and arms get activated. If you are frustrated, you might get the urge to yell. Some of these action urges are associated with connection and protection states. For example, if you are very activated and angry, you may have an action urge to fight. If you are activated and afraid, you might have an urge to run. Learning to be with sensations and notice them means being with and noticing the action urges that may accompany them. As you feel sensations, take time to notice any action urges.

Trait #5: Sensations arise and pass

Sensations are impermanent: they arise and pass. Perhaps this is the most important characteristic of sensations to remember. Grabovac *et al.* (2011) consider this realization central to wellbeing. As you notice sensations, notice their impermanence, their transience. They sometimes feel like a wave, coming into awareness, increasing in intensity, and then slowly receding. Yoga is the ideal practice for this type of noticing. Through each pose and, more broadly, through the sequence of poses, the yoga student will experience many different sensations. For each one, the student can practice awareness, noticing its qualities and working with the posture and breath to be with the sensations. Some sensations might suggest a need for a yoga block for support, others might call for a steady breath. Still others, despite their intensity and associated action urge, would be best served simply by being with them as they arise and pass.

> **Journal Prompt.** Choose a yoga pose and hold the pose for 60–90 seconds. As you hold the pose, orient your awareness on one sensation. Consider what information this sensation is offering. If it could speak, what would it say? How would you describe the sensation (size, shape, texture, etc.)? Does it feel comfortable, uncomfortable, or neutral? Does this sensation have an action urge? What is it? Does the sensation change? Increase in intensity? Do you notice qualities of impermanence—arising and passing? Write down what you noticed.

Not Sensation Seeking

Noticing sensations is not the same thing as sensation seeking. When you emphasize sensations as a yoga teacher, it is important to emphasize curiosity, observation, and acceptance. Students can sometimes misunderstand the experiencing of intense sensations as a goal. They speak to us about our inner world and our bodies. Sensations arise and pass. In this way, there are times when they are not present, and this is okay. Consider being hungry and full. There are also times when you are not either. This is not an on-demand process. If experiencing intense sensations becomes the goal of yoga, the student loses the *being with* quality of yoga practice. This can turn into yet another way that goal seeking overtakes the yoga. It is not much different than seeking the perfect version of a pose.

Sensations, Hypermobility, and Dissociation

It is important to talk about the experience of wanting but not being able to feel or perceive sensations. Two pertinent conditions that are associated with this experience are hypermobility and dissociation.

Yoga students with hypermobility (the condition of having a significantly broader range of motion than most people) may not feel sensations in the same ways that others do. When seeking sensations, or *feeling something*, they are at risk of over-stretching connective tissues and injury. It is important to cue for keeping a slight bend in the joints and to notice sensations in the belly of the muscles, skin, and overall viscera, rather than seeking a sensation in the joints or at the full expression of a pose.

Dissociation—feeling detached or disconnected from your body, the environment and people around you—is something we all experience. It is a way that your brain attempts to manage too much stress or trauma. In its mildest form, it is a coping strategy that most of us use. In extremes, such as what can occur with a traumatizing experience, a person may feel nothing at all—no sensations, no connection to others, and no sense of connection with the world. In this case, mental health support is encouraged.

You may teach yoga students who report feeling nothing. They may be hypermobile. They may be dissociating. There may be nothing to feel in the moment. Encourage your students to notice what is there, even if that is nothing. For students who regularly report the lack of feeling-sensations, or for whom you have become concerned that they seem to be sensation seeking to the point of risk, consider your scope of practice and refer for mental health treatment or physical therapy support.

Conclusion

Now that you are familiar with the five key traits of sensations, you are prepared to learn more about the experience of sensations and their role in the processing of emotions. Consider the questions below. Make sure you can describe the five traits of sensations and how sensations are experienced uniquely from person to person. Last, begin a contemplation on the powerful role that sensations play in your yoga teaching and your students' experiences as they practice, and its relation to being trauma-informed and responsive.

TEACHER TRAINING DISCUSSION QUESTIONS

1. Describe the five traits of sensations.

2. "There is no universal relationship between safety and sensations that can be applied to all people." What does this mean?

3. In what ways can learning about sensations support your work as a TIR yoga teacher?

CHAPTER 8

Sensations as Communication—Physiology, Emotions, Memories, and State Activation

prakâȃa-kriyâ-sthiti-ȃîlaä bhûtendriyâtmakaä
bhogâpavargârthaä dëȃyam

Yoga Sutra II:18

Things seen have as their property manifestation, action, inertia [sensation qualities and associated action urges]. They form the basis of the elements and the sense-powers. They make for experience [being with and working with] and for liberation [freedom from suffering].

Charles Johnston (1912)

Sensations are in and of themselves experiences. They arise, pass, and can be experienced externally, physically, and psychologically. Sensations are pertinent to trauma-informed and responsive (TIR) yoga teaching. They communicate our (1) external experiences, (2) physiological processes and experiences, (3) physiological aspects of emotions, (4) physical memories, and (5) in-the-moment state activation. Taken together, we can say sensations are experiences, in and of themselves, *and* they communicate experiences our bodies are having to us. In yoga, we learn to both experience and listen to our sensations. As TIR yoga teachers, we support our students as they learn to both experience and listen to their sensations. This chapter will explore sensations from the perspective of their communication to us.

> **TIR PRINCIPLE: SENSATIONS ARE EXPERIENCES AND COMMUNICATIONS**
> Sensations are experiences that arise and pass that tell us about our embodied experiences.

1. Sensations Tell Us About Our External Experiences

You might recall from elementary school that your sensations include sight, sound, touch, smell, and taste. Your five senses—a large part of your *exteroceptive awareness*—provide information about the outside world (Cook-Cottone, 2023). In yoga, this might be your feet and hands pressing into your mat, the resonance of a singing bowl's sound waves as they move through your body and eardrums, or the smell of incense encountered walking into your studio. You can see where the other students are in the room, where the exits are, or if someone is moving towards you in a way that doesn't seem safe or that seems like a pleasant greeting. Often, when thinking about sensations, it is our five senses we immediately call to mind.

2. Sensations Tell Us About Our Physiological Experiences

Some sensations help you know what is going on inside your body and are associated with *interoceptive awareness* (Cook-Cottone, 2023). These sensations inform you of hunger, thirst, tiredness, and more, including the state of your muscles and joints (e.g., muscle fatigue, joint pain). It is the pain in your knees during Camel Pose (*Ustrasana*) that reminds you to place a towel under your knees or fold your yoga mat over for support.

3. Sensations Tell Us About Our Physiological Aspects of Emotions

Emotions are experienced as physiological sensations, feeling-based thoughts, and action urges (or impulses to take feeling-based actions). Focusing on the physiological sensations that accompany emotions, Lauri Nummenmaa and colleagues (2014) published a groundbreaking study. Researchers induced feeling states in participants and then asked each participant to use a human figure drawing to indicate where they sensed activity felt stronger and faster and/or weaker and slower. Results representing emotional sadness are depicted in Figure 8.1. When experiencing sadness, on average, participants felt activation in regions of the face and across the chest with deactivation in their arms, pelvis, and legs. Consider the feeling-sensations you notice when you are experiencing an emotion. Perhaps you feel a tingle in your belly when you feel anxious, a deep, heavy feeling around your heart with grief, or the expansion in your chest with joy. Anytime you are working with the body, as we do in yoga, your students will be activating regions of their bodies in which they experience feeling-sensations. In *Savasana*, a student may have their hands on their chest, noticing the slow beat of their heart, and perhaps something more. It is not uncommon for a remembered trace of sadness, joy, or grief to move through this region, where these emotions are so often experienced.

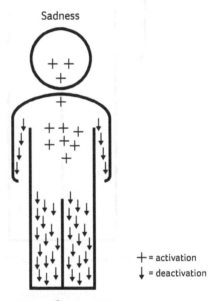

FIGURE 8.1 SADNESS

> **Journal Prompt.** Figure 8.2 is an outline of a body. The next time you experience an emotion, notice the feeling-sensations present in your body. Pause and take a moment to breathe, just noticing the sensations. When you are ready, use colors or the activation (+) and deactivation (↓) symbols to illustrate the feeling-sensations you notice in your body. This can be a fun exploration over time. You might want to do this in a separate journal—jot down the feeling and the date and a little about the circumstances.

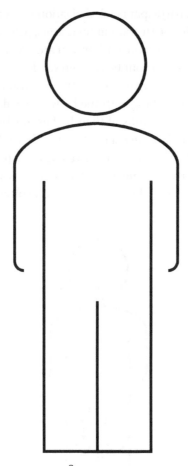

FIGURE 8.2 HUMAN FIGURE

Table 8.1 shows the findings of Nummenmaa *et al.*'s (2014) study. It can be interesting to compare your drawings to what was observed across participants in their research. You may notice many of the activation patterns occur within the ventral vagal area, where we communicate with each other in relationships (head, arms, hands, upper torso). Emotions are meant to communicate to you and others what you are experiencing. You might also notice that emotions tend to be mobilizing or immobilizing.

A student shared with me (CCC) that she noticed that anger, fear, and love all activated the area around her heart. She reflected on this and then shared that she now realized that if she did not acknowledge and feel the anger and fear in her life so that it could move through, she might not notice all of the love that is present. They all take up the space of the heart. Something to think about, isn't it?

Table 8.1 Nummenmaa et al.'s Body Maps of Emotion Patterns of Activation and Deactivation

Ventral Vagal Areas

Feeling	Anger	Fear	Anxiety	Happiness	Sadness	Depression	Shame	Love
Head	++++	++	+	+++	+	↓↓	+++	+++
Neck/throat	+++	++	++	++	+	↓↓	++	+++
Shoulders	+++	+	n	++	↓	↓↓↓	n	++
Upper arms	+++	+	n	+++	↓	↓↓↓	↓	++
Lower arms	+++	+	n	+++	↓↓	↓↓↓	↓	++
Hands	++++	++	n	+++	↓	↓↓	n	++
Chest/heart	++++	+++	+++	++++	++	n	++	+++
Upper abdomen	++	+	++	+++	+	n	+	++

Dorsal Vagal Areas

Feeling	Anger	Fear	Anxiety	Happiness	Sadness	Depression	Shame	Love
Lower abdomen	n	+	+	++	n	n	+	+++
Hips/pelvis	n	n	n	+	↓↓	↓	n	+++
Upper legs	+	+	↓↓	++	↓↓	↓↓↓	↓	++
Lower legs	+	+	↓↓	++	↓↓	↓↓↓	↓	+
Feet	+	+	↓↓	++	↓↓↓	↓↓↓↓	↓↓	+

n = neutral; + mild activation; ++ moderate activation; +++ strong activation; ++++ very strong activation; ↓ mild deactivation; ↓↓ moderate deactivation; ↓↓↓ strong deactivation; ↓↓↓↓ very strong deactivation

(Nummenmaa et al., 2014)

Journal Prompt. How might feeling-sensations play a role in how a student experiences a yoga class? What might you notice if a student is struggling with grief or depression? What might you notice in a student who just received a work promotion before class? What might you notice in a student waiting to get medical test results? How might considering feeling-sensations shift your yoga teaching?

4. Sensations Tell Us About Our Physical Aspects of Memories

Like emotions, memories are experienced in complex ways (Cook-Cottone, 2023). We think of memories almost like a story with its narrative replaying in our heads. Sometimes we experience the feelings and feeling-sensations associated with the memory. Importantly, our bodies are also part of our remembering system. Bessel van der Kolk's (2014) best-selling book *The Body Keeps the Score: Brain, Mind, and Body in the Healing of Trauma* changed the way clinicians think about trauma and trauma memories, highlighting the value of yoga and relationships in the healing process. You might notice your muscles begin tensing and your heart rate increases when bringing a stressful experience to mind. This is a top-down process: you remember the story in your head as thoughts (top), then feel it activate your body (down). Consider that tensing or releasing your muscles in a certain way, the position of your body, and the physiological state you are in can also activate memories. This is a bottom-up process. Your body experiences sensations (bottom) which triggers a cognitive memory (top). This means that in any class, in any pose, your yoga students may be triggering or activating difficult memories.

> To illustrate, Shannon (he/him) was sexually abused as a child. His stepfather abused him while everyone was in bed and asleep. He is in therapy and working on his wellbeing. Yoga is an important part of his work. He has not told the teacher in his neighborhood studio about his past. Despite his work and the passage of many years, Shannon still has difficulty with *Savasana*. It activates the memory of lying in bed afraid of his stepfather. His muscles tense, his heart begins to race, and sometimes he begins sweating. He feels shaky and overwhelmed. He is working on being able to close his eyes and stay in *Savasana* for one minute before he rolls up his mat and leaves. Each week, he makes a little more progress. He was thrilled last week because he made it to 90 seconds with his eyes closed.

SENSATIONS AS COMMUNICATION

Journal Prompt. How does it feel to have a student leave, or fidget, during *Savasana*? In what ways does considering a possible trauma history shift your response?

5. Sensations Tell Us About Our State Activation

Interoceptive sensations let you know what state you might be in (think back to the polyvagal theory): active engagement, fight or flight, shutdown—via activation indicators such as heart and breath rates and muscle tension. Each of the other types of sensations can affect your state activation level (Cook-Cottone, 2023).

> For example, during yoga, when George (he/him) notices his heart rate increasing, he often feels triggered and afraid. He rates himself a 5 or 6 on the self-regulation scale. He is a veteran and associates his increased heart rate with danger since his deployment. He is working on staying present and aware, simply breathing gently and reminding himself he is safe right here and right now. This can quickly get him moving toward a rating of 4. Sometimes, however, his increased heart rate triggers images and memories from the war, sending him into fight or flight (a rating of 7 or 8 and escalating). In yoga class, he often digs into about 20 push-ups to get a hold of himself. This gets him back to a 6 and moving in the right direction toward a 5.

> Sky (she/her) has been diagnosed with depression and has a history of trauma, a sexual assault in college. She has been attending yoga classes two or three times a week as recommended by her therapist. Her TIR yoga teacher taught her about practicing the PAUSE whenever she needed or wanted to during class (see box below and Chapter 3). Sky has noticed she is beginning to feel her feelings again. Recently, when in Dancer Pose (*Natarajasana*), she felt an opening across her chest and was feeling something like happiness and joy. It was all a bit overwhelming: her heart rate increased, her breath became shallow, and her self-regulation scale rating quickly went from a 4 to a 7. She grounded both feet on her mat and stood in Mountain Pose (*Tadasana*) for three gentle belly breaths and then took a Forward Fold. She joined the class for the second side of Dancer Pose (*Natarajasana*) at a 5 and holding steady with a deeply grounded foot and focusing on her breath.

> **PRACTICING THE PAUSE**
> Any time, any place, and for any reason, you can always PAUSE. Pause = stop what you are doing, A = assess how you are and what you need, and USE = use your resources.

Although we are all different in how we experience sensations, knowing what each state activation level feels like in your body is the first step in knowing how they might feel for someone else. In Table 8.2, document the body sensations you notice in yourself when you are in each state. If this is difficult, begin by taking a week or two to notice your body when you are in different embodied states. You might jot notes in your phone to help you complete the table. Be sure to include breath rate, the nature of the breath (smooth, halting, etc.), heart rate, areas of muscle tension and release, what you notice in your abdomen, along with sweat and temperature of the body. As you increase your own ability to recognize shifts in your body across the various embodied states, you will also become better at noticing these same shifts in your yoga students (Cook-Cottone, 2023).

Table 8.2 Nervous System Self-Regulation Scale and Embodied States

How Regulated Are You?

Regulated ← 1 2 3 4 5 6 7 8 9 10 → Dysregulated

Restful • Calm • Engaged • Growing • Challenged • Fight/Flight • Freeze • Overwhelmed

Embodied State	Accompanying Body Sensations
Restful	
Calm	
Engaged	
Growing	
Challenged	

SENSATIONS AS COMMUNICATION

↓ Outside of the Window of Tolerance ↓	
Fight/Flight	
Freeze	
Overwhelmed/Shutdown	

Journal Prompt. What did you notice as you explored the sensations associated with the various states? Note, for some people, this process can be difficult. It can take practice to tune into your sensations. It can be overwhelming or you might not feel anything. Remember that all experiences are welcome and valid. If you felt a lot, too much, or nothing, describe what that was like for you.

Conclusion

Sensations communicate to us about a variety of embodied experiences. Discerning the different communicative role of emotions can be very helpful as you and your yoga students work on relationships with your bodies. Now that you have reviewed the key traits of sensations and their role in communicating embodied experiences, you are ready to dig deeper into the role sensations play in self-regulation.

TEACHER TRAINING DISCUSSION QUESTIONS

1. Explain what it means to say that sensations are both experiences in and of themselves and communications associated with our embodied selves.
2. What are the embodied experiences about which sensations communicate to us?
3. In what ways are sensations associated with feelings?
4. How is state activation different from having an emotion? How is it the same?
5. Is it okay to struggle to feel sensations, not feel sensations, or feel a bit overwhelmed by sensations?

6. Why is it helpful, for your yoga teaching, for you to explore how sensations are experienced in your body?

7. Why might it be important for the TIR teaching of yoga to be aware of the different embodied experiences about which sensations are communicating?

CHAPTER 9

Sensations and Self-Regulation

yogaå citta-vëtti-nirodhaï

Yoga Sutra 1:2

Union, spiritual consciousness [yoga], is gained through control of the versatile psychic nature [stilling of the mind].

Charles Johnston (1912)

Patanjali, an ancient sage of yoga, states that the goal of yoga in yoga sutra 1:2 is decreasing the fluctuations, or thought waves, of the mind (Desikachar, 1995; Prabhavananda & Isherwood, 2007). This makes so much sense to anyone who practices regularly. There is nothing like a deeply connected yoga practice to calm the body and still the mind. It is easy to read this sutra without fully appreciating the depths of what is being said. This sutra speaks to the power of embodied practices in the regulation of the nervous system. In his interpretation of the sutras, T. K. V. Desikachar (1995) describes yoga as a process for tying the strands of the mind together, a process we now refer to as neurological integration. This form of self-regulation referenced in the sutras and experienced in your practice is called *embodied self-regulation* (Cook-Cottone, 2015). It is distinct from Western formulations of self-regulation focusing on cognitive or thinking processes used to accomplish goals or manage thoughts and feelings (Cook-Cottone, 2015; Karoly, 1993). Embodied self-regulation is about learning, growing, integrating, and healing as an active process occurring within the doing, the practice. It is more formally defined as the "integration of mind and body, through active practice as you work toward balanced and sustainable self-mastery within the context of attunement within the self and among others" (Cook-Cottone, 2015, p. 9).

As trauma-informed and responsive (TIR) yoga teachers, part of our role is to teach our students the yoga skills and practices to support their healing, growth, and embodied self-regulation in ways that do not set them back, increase dysregulation, and/or get in the way of the natural growth and healing processes. This process begins by working with students exactly where they are, increasing their awareness, and carefully scaffolding new skills on previously mastered, practiced skills. Through attuned and responsive practice, the yoga student is able "to attain what was previously unattainable" (Desikachar, 1995, p. 5). This chapter will explore some ways in which that is done.

> **TIR PRINCIPLE:** MEET THE STUDENT EXACTLY WHERE THEY ARE
>
> Trauma-informed and responsive yoga meets the yoga student exactly where they are with non-judgment, loving-kindness, and carefully scaffolded instruction.

Ahimsa and Satya and Embodied Self-Regulation

Yoga as a pathway to embodied self-regulation begins with the first two yamas from the yoga sutras—*ahimsa and satya*. The yamas are the first limb of yoga in the eight-limb path, and are often thought of as the disciplines or restraints that support the relationship between an individual and the outside world (Desikachar, 1995; Ranganathan, 2008). They are the rules of moral conduct. The first, ahimsa, refers to non-harming, a central concept of TIR yoga teaching. According to Ranganathan (2008), ahimsa is the most important yama, serving as the master moral principle to be followed by both word and deed. The yamas that follow can all be understood as ways of carrying out non-harmfulness (Ranganathan, 2008). In his interpretation of the sutras, Desikachar (1995) states that ahimsa refers to *more than* the absence of violence. It means kindness, friendliness, and a thoughtful consideration of and attention to others. In this way, yoga is inherently trauma-informed and responsive, and that is why it is the teaching of yoga that is the focus of our work (rather than yoga itself).

The second, *satya*, refers to truthfulness, to speak and act from an honest relationship with the present moment, yourself, and others. Ahimsa cannot happen without satya. Applied specifically to the teaching of yoga, we cannot safely teach yoga (honoring ahimsa) without knowing the truth about the effects of postures and practices and the physiological, emotional, and cognitive states of our students. For example, we must first know the shoulder's specific range of motion before encouraging a student to go further. What would be a lovely stretch for one shoulder can be a muscle-pulling, joint-damaging stretch for another. To illustrate further, a vigorous vinyasa practice might be exactly what one person needs, yet overwhelming and stressful for another. To be a TIR yoga teacher, you must be committed to being aware, knowing your yoga students, and how that practice affects your students. Otherwise, you are at high risk for doing harm.

Truth, satya, can be found in our ability to be aware of, experience, and respond to our sensations. Our bodies communicate the state of our physiological and emotional selves, and the nature of our connection to the outside world through sensations. You will know your shoulder is injured as a sharp pain shoots from your shoulder to your neck in *Chaturanga Dandasana* (Half Plank Pose). You will know how hungry you are when your stomach grumbles and a little ache begins to nag at you. Your throat and mouth signal thirst. A heaviness in your chest signals grief and a lightness in your heart area signals joy. You get a gut feeling when someone feels unsafe. You quickly draw your hand away as you feel pain when a surface is too hot. You lean in to snuggle your pet, feeling the warmth and familiarity of their fur.

Understanding and connecting to sensations is the foundation of self-knowledge, your truth. In this way, sensations are foundational in the practice of non-harming. We learn we can trust our bodies as a source of knowing how we are, what drives us, and ultimately who we are. When we know who we are, our actions and words come from an integrated and intentional experience of self. Knowing your truth, you can begin to trust yourself, and this is the pathway to being trustworthy.

Sensations and the Self-Regulatory Feedback Loop

With all of the different functions of sensations, it is a lot for a human nervous system to sort out. It is through our interoception and exteroception of sensations that the connection and protection processes arise. To become competent at embodied self-regulation, it can be very helpful to become competent at noticing, being with, and working with your sensations. Like Sky in the case example above, noticing your sensations and activation levels, you and your yoga students can implement practices like PAUSE.

As you learn more about the key traits of sensations (sensations as experiences and modes of embodied communication and information associated with your physiological states), the self-regulation scale becomes increasingly more meaningful and helpful (see Figure 9.1). When within one's window of tolerance, there is greater access to both connection with self and others and self-regulation. In fact, the access to connection with self and others supports self-regulation. Conversely, when you or your yoga students are outside of your window of tolerance, the body and mind become protective, offering limited access to self-regulation. The reactive parts of the brain are preferentially activated (e.g., the limbic system), and the parts of the brain helpful in self-regulation (e.g., the frontal cortex) are much less likely to be engaged. Feelings are experienced as driving, dysregulated somatic experiences. Thoughts can become mirrors of the reactive state (e.g., "I am not safe" and "I am overwhelmed"), rather than a pathway for noticing and self-regulation (e.g., "I am noticing reactivity" and "I need to ground my feet and breathe"). In this state, others are likely seen as the threat. It is our relationship with our sensations that will help us assess our states and respond effectively, increasing the chance we will stay in or quickly return to our window of tolerance.

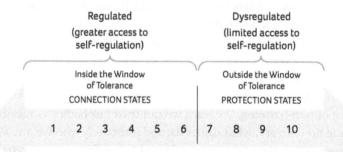

FIGURE 9.1 ENHANCED SELF-REGULATION SCALE—ACCESS TO SELF-REGULATION, WINDOW OF TOLERANCE, AND CONNECTION AND PROTECTION STATES

It can be helpful to break the process down from the first experience of a sensation through the process of detection and state activation. As illustrated in Figure 9.2, sensations can arise from any of the key sensation sources. You notice or become aware of the sensations through either interoception or exteroception. You instantaneously and automatically make an assessment of the safety or threat associated with the sensations that you notice (i.e., neuroception). In accordance with the neuroceptive assessment, your nervous system either moves toward a protective and reactive state or an engaged and connected state.

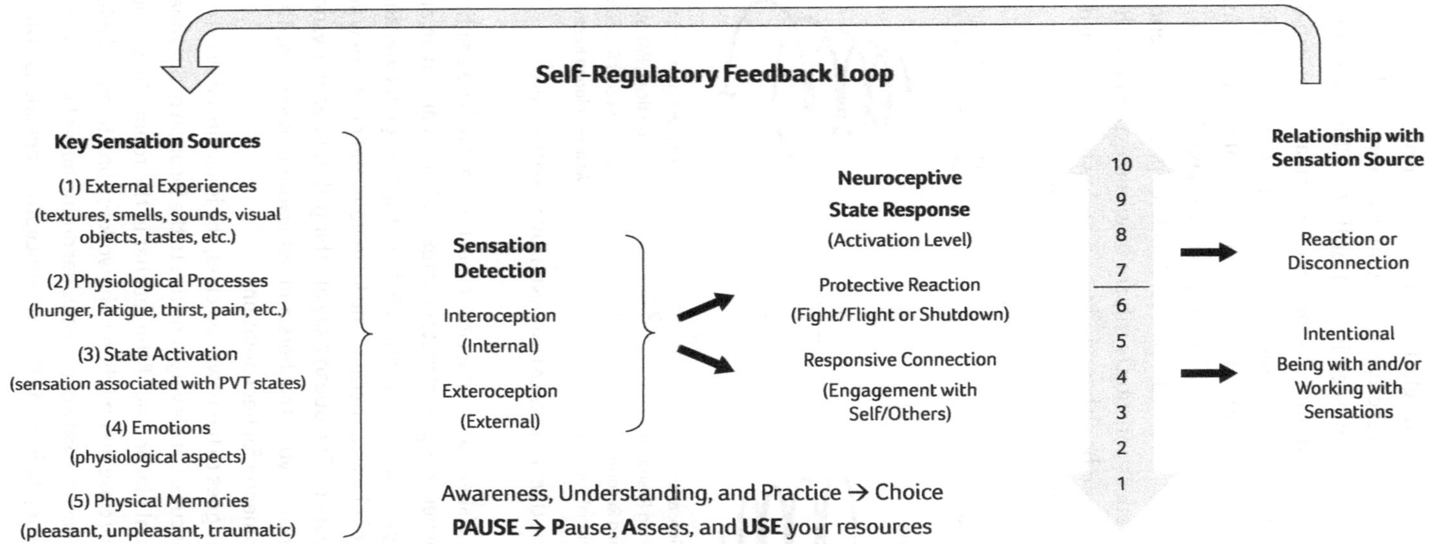

Self-Regulatory Feedback Loop

Key Sensation Sources

(1) External Experiences
(textures, smells, sounds, visual objects, tastes, etc.)

(2) Physiological Processes
(hunger, fatigue, thirst, pain, etc.)

(3) State Activation
(sensation associated with PVT states)

(4) Emotions
(physiological aspects)

(5) Physical Memories
(pleasant, unpleasant, traumatic)

Sensation Detection

Interoception (Internal)

Exteroception (External)

Neuroceptive State Response
(Activation Level)

Protective Reaction
(Fight/Flight or Shutdown)

Responsive Connection
(Engagement with Self/Others)

10
9
8
7
6
5
4
3
2
1

Relationship with Sensation Source

Reaction or Disconnection

Intentional Being with and/or Working with Sensations

Awareness, Understanding, and Practice → Choice
PAUSE → **Pause, Assess,** and **USE** your resources

FIGURE 9.2 SENSATIONS AND THE SELF-REGULATORY FEEDBACK LOOP
(Informed by Cook-Cottone, 2023; Dana, 2020, Porges, 2021)

This, in turn, informs your relationship with the original sensation. If you are in a protective and reactive state, you are more likely to respond in reactions of disconnection seen in fight or flight. This is what happens to George (see case example above) sometimes. If you are in or can down-regulate into an engaged and connected state, you are more likely to intentionally be with and/or work with the experience of the sensation. This is what happens when George does his push-ups and Sky (above) practices PAUSE. This process is considered a feedback loop. Your current state and intentional awareness constantly inform how you experience the next set of sensations. You can be either winding up or down-regulating depending on your awareness and ability to use your resources (see Figure 9.3).

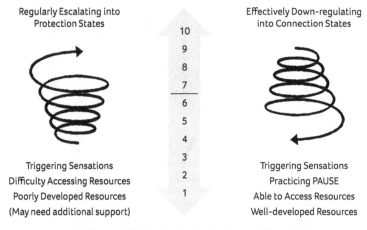

FIGURE 9.3 ESCALATING AND DOWN-REGULATING

> Consider Sara (she/her). A small muscle in the front of Sara's right shoulder was injured when a yoga instructor overextended her arm in an attempt to provide a physical assist. The injury led to a trip to urgent care, an MRI, and eight weeks of physical therapy. She loves yoga and finds a new yoga class and a new teacher. She doesn't say anything about her injury, not feeling entirely trusting of yoga teachers and not wanting to seem as though she is blaming someone for her condition.
>
> When she goes to her new yoga class, she is sensitized to exteroceptive sensations or cues. Sara is very sensitive to the location of the yoga instructor—the visual placement of the teacher in the room, the sound of their voice, and how close they might be. She works on breathing and relaxing into poses. She is keenly aware of her shoulder during poses like Downward-Facing Dog Pose and Side Plank Pose (interoceptive sensations). During these

SENSATIONS AND SELF-REGULATION

poses, she can feel her breath shorten and speed up, and she experiences an increase of muscle tension across her whole body as her body warns her that these poses (and the yoga teacher) might not be safe (neuroception). This increased muscle tension and shallow and quick breathing sometimes activate pain receptors around her injury. Sara can often feel herself getting worked up and defensive. She moves from a 4 or 5 on the self-regulation scale to a 7. In a flight reaction, her thoughts are "I can't do this." At a certain point, in the middle of class, she becomes so upset that she rolls up her mat and heads home in tears (she's at an 8). Sara has not yet developed tools or resources to manage the escalating states of her body. She has never learned how to practice PAUSE or anything like it. It takes her half of the day to down-regulate into an engaged and connected state. Worse, she engages in negative self-talk, blaming herself for over-reacting.

Journal Prompt. If you were Sara's new yoga teacher, what would you notice? You might notice her being careful when doing poses on her right side. Despite your commitment to checking in with students, Sara tells you nothing. You might notice her breath rate, her face flushing—what else? What does it feel like when she walks out of your class? How can you empower her, give her voice and choice?

Conclusion

In yoga, we get a chance to practice feeling, exploring, and responding to sensations and emotions. It is empowering and very challenging. We get a chance to decide if we will just experience them or act on them. In the accepting and nurturing space of a yoga class (especially a trauma-informed and responsive space), we get the chance to experience all of this. Further, as a TIR yoga teacher, the more competence you have in being with and working with your emotions, the more sensitive and attuned you will be with your students. Yoga is always inviting us to feel, which is a complicated and potentially overwhelming process. Helping students develop awareness, understanding, and choice around their sensations will help them meet yoga's invitation to feel with grounded feet, a soft open heart, and steady breath.

TEACHER TRAINING DISCUSSION QUESTIONS

1. How do the concepts of ahimsa and satya relate to TIR teaching?

2. Why is knowing yourself and being trustworthy so important when teaching yoga?

3. Why is the ability to be with discomfort critical to growth and healing?

4. Describe the association between state activation (number on the self-regulation scale), connection and protection states, and access to self-regulation.

5. What role does the forward or upward spiral play in practicing and teaching yoga? How does knowing about these concepts help us be trauma-informed and responsive?

PART III

TRAUMA-INFORMED AND RESPONSIVE COMMUNICATION

CHAPTER 10

Communication Basics— Mindful and Heartful Listening

*maitrî-karuñâ-muditopekæâñââ sukha-duïkha-
puñyâpuñya-viæayâñââ bhâvanâtaâ citta-prasâdanam*

Yoga Sutra 1:33

Mentality brightens, and gets to be of a serene disposition and good humour, when one takes on an attitude of friendliness towards the pleasant, of compassion for those who suffer, of joy for the meritorious, and of equanimity towards the unmeritorious.

Shyam Ranganathan (2008)

Communication is the practice of using our words and body to connect with others, allowing others to know our experiences, feelings, and thoughts and for us to receive the same from others. Our communication is ultimately who we are to our students. It is how they know us. Consider that when you communicate as a yoga teacher to yoga students, you are speaking within the context of a power differential. The potential impact of your words is more substantial than you might realize. Even if you do not feel powerful, your position is one of power in relation to your students. As a trauma-informed and responsive (TIR) yoga teacher, it is important that you develop a deep awareness of what you are saying and to remember how much what you say matters.

Your words are powerful. They can create connections (support ventral vagal states) or move people into defensive protection (sympathetic and overwhelmed dorsal states). Your use of words and language is a practice much like yoga, filled with and informed by your mindful awareness, intentions, and commitment to non-harming, truth, compassion, and loving-kindness. Your words are a bridge from you and your embodied knowledge of yoga to your students. Your words help develop a sense of safety, trustworthiness, support, mutuality, empowerment, and voice. When communicated effectively, your words facilitate connection and support students' personal and unique journeys through practice, discovery, and the embodiment of yoga. More broadly, your words and how they are used create the atmosphere within which your yoga sessions and classes are experienced. This includes the words used with your students. It also includes how you speak to yourself (your inner dialogue), fellow yoga teachers, staff, and associates within your business or organization.

The next three chapters will address how you can effectively use words to support connection states, while reducing risk of harm. This chapter will focus on communication with others—mindful and heartful listening. In the final two chapters on communication, you will explore nonviolent communication, content warnings, and microaggressions.

> **TIR PRINCIPLE:** HUMANS HAVE A FUNDAMENTAL NEED TO BE SEEN AND HEARD
> Learn and practice mindful and heartful listening in which seeing and hearing are prioritized over being right and problem solving.

TIR PRACTICE: MINDFUL LISTENING

Perhaps the most misunderstood aspect of communicating effectively is the focus on the right words to say. In reality, the most important aspect of communicating effectively is listening. Listening is a core feature of a connection state. There are two very helpful listening practices that should be core content for all yoga teacher trainings: mindful and heartful listening. These practices are good for day-to-day listening and can be quite helpful when someone is having a difficult time and needing to be seen and heard.

Mindful listening is the practice of being mindfully present and listening to another with curiosity, openness, and loving-kindness. You do not listen so that you can respond effectively. You listen to truly see and hear another human. This is a powerful practice. To be seen and heard are two fundamental needs of human beings.

Begin the practice ensuring you and your partner (the person to whom you are listening) are seated comfortably and feel grounded and supported. Take a moment and breathe several breath cycles with an extended exhale (in 1, 2, 3, 4 and out 1, 2, 3, 4, 5). Next, your partner simply shares what they are thinking, an experience they've had, anything they'd like to say. You simply listen. Here, your partner and their words are the object of your attention. You add gestures showing you are present and listening such as nodding, making eye contact, and offering a half-smile. You do not speak, ask questions, or clarify. Your goal is to deeply listen—that is all. When they are finished, you can simply thank them for sharing their experience with you. You can also share back the content of what you heard, without adding any interpretations, inferences, analysis, or solutions. You might say "What I heard you say was..." or simply summarize their sharing.

For example, your partner (they/them) shares a story about walking into the yoga space to teach a class and finding yoga mats and blocks not put away, incense ashes on the counter, and the bathroom baskets full of garbage. As a result, they had to pick up rather than get centered and prepared for class. You might say, "When you got to the studio, things were a mess and you were not able to prepare for class." Feeling seen and heard, your partner will often continue sharing their experience. "Yes, and I was scattered and ungrounded as I started the class." You would add in summary form, "It affected your teaching." You do not give them advice about how they might have started class with a grounding pose and breaths (even if that is a great idea). You simply listen and reflect. They might add, "It did, and then I realized, I know what to do. I can do a grounding pose, have us all take deep breaths together... It all worked out in the end. But what a day." Listening, you respond, "You noticed what was needed and turned things around. Your own practice helped you know what to do." Imagine what might have been missed if the listener tried to fix, offer advice, or interject.

Your partner will respond if they meant or said something different. It's okay if they do. This feedback will help you improve your skills. Ultimately, what matters is that you are truly trying to hear what they are sharing (it's about them), which is much better than worrying about being a perfect listener or the best advice giver (it's about you).

Journal Prompt. What does it feel like to listen mindfully? Is it difficult for you not to interject, interpret, analyze, or solve problems? What does it feel like to make your listening about the other person and not about you and your response? How might your urges to speak, interpret, analyze, or fix get in the way of truly hearing someone? What other options or responses can you explore instead? How might you integrate this practice into your life?

TIR PRACTICE: HEARTFUL LISTENING

Heartful listening is an extension of mindful listening. In heartful listening, your focus is on the feelings and needs present in the sharing. When someone is experiencing a difficult feeling, facilitating a connection state by heartfully listening can be very helpful. As with mindful listening, this is not an analysis or interpretation. Rather, it is deeply listening to what the person is telling you about their felt experience. It can be very helpful to notice your own body, your *felt sense*, as they tell the story. Our nervous systems are designed to pick up on the emotional states of others. As social mammals, we are hard-wired to have empathy for one another.

As you practice heartful listening, ensure you are grounded in your seat (or on your feet) and in an open and receptive position (e.g., your arms are by your sides or hands gently resting on your lap, not crossed in front of your chest). Your chest or heart area is open, and you have a soft gaze as you listen. As your partner speaks, ask yourself, "What is this person feeling?" Notice their tone of voice, pace of speech, body language, and eyes as they speak. Notice any sensations arising in your own body as they tell their story, such as the sensation of tears coming to your eyes and aches or heaviness in your belly, a tightening or loosening of contractions in your belly or chest, the beating of your heart, breath rate, and activation of the arms, shoulders, or muscles in the face. Then label what you are noticing and feeling. For example, is it sadness, anger, fear, regret, frustration, or joy? When they have finished sharing, you might say "What I heard you feel was…" or, more informally, "You felt…"

For example, your friend (they/them) is telling you about the yoga studio, the mess, and having to teach class. They are agitated, hyped up, and their voice is high pitched and shaky. Their arms are animated, and you notice a wateriness in their eyes. They say, "I walked into the studio, and I was shocked. There were mats lying across the floor, blocks in a pile by the desk, incense ashes on the desk, and the garbage was full. I felt sad that someone would leave the studio this way, knowing I had class. I had to pick it all up and try to get myself settled for class. It was overwhelming." As a heartful listener, you might say, "The whole thing was overwhelming. You were shocked and discouraged." The focus of your response is the feeling, not the details. Your partner might clarify, "Yeah, I was overwhelmed. And to be honest, I was more sad than shocked." In this case, your response allowed them to get clear on their feelings.

As with mindful listening, the power of heartful listening is your effort to truly see and hear the experience of another. Take time to practice as you connect with your students, peers, and loved ones. Consider practicing both types of listening in your teacher training or workshops. As you do, take time to notice how these types of listening affect your relationships.

Journal Prompt. What does it feel like to heartfully listen to others? Is it difficult to orient simply on the emotional experience? What is it like to use your own felt sense to better understand others? What have you noticed in others when you are listening in this way?

Conclusion

So much of what we do as yoga teachers is directing, teaching, suggesting, and other forms of advising our yoga students. This chapter is here to remind you that it is critical for you to simply make space for your student, beginning with listening more than talking. Mindful and heartfelt listening gives you two tools for helping students feel seen and heard. They are TIR practices as they highlight agency and self-determination and honor the experience of the other person speaking.

TEACHER TRAINING DISCUSSION QUESTIONS

1. How is mindful and heartful listening different from how you typically communicate with others?

2. What (if anything) is difficult about the process?

3. In what ways might increasing your mindful and heartful listening practice affect your relationships with your yoga students?

CHAPTER 11

Nonviolent Communication and Conflict

vastu-sâmye citta-bhedât tayor vibhaktaï panthâï

Yoga Sutra IV:15

The paths of material things and of states of consciousness are distinct, as is manifest from the fact that the same object may produce different impressions in different minds.

Charles Johnston (1912)

Nonviolent communication can create a safer environment within which you offer yoga sessions or classes. It is a way of resolving conflicts that emphasizes relationships, personal needs, and empathy (Rosenberg, 2012). Nonviolent communication supports connection, or ventral vagal states, rather than defensive protection states such as fight, flight, and shutdown. Instead of focusing on what we want out of the conflict, the focus is on creating conditions in which everyone's needs might be met: connection (Rosenberg, 2012). Nonviolent communication supports the trauma-informed values of trustworthiness, transparency, peer support, collaboration, mutuality, empowerment, voice, and choice.

How you communicate with others outside of yoga sessions matters. Aligned with the practice of ahimsa, nonviolent communication begins with awareness. In their book *What We Say Matters: Practicing Nonviolent Communication*, Judith Hanson Lasater and Ike Lasater (2022) explain that nonviolent communication is "first about self-awareness and then about empathy for self and others" (p. xv). Your ongoing yoga practice and work in previous chapters prepares you for the level of awareness you need to communicate clearly and nonviolently.

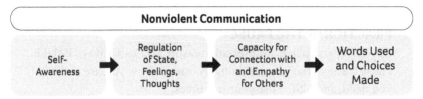

FIGURE 11.1 NONVIOLENT COMMUNICATION

Nonviolent communication, a ventral vagal practice, is fundamentally about an underlying intention to connect with ourselves and then to others (Lasater & Lasater, 2022). When practicing nonviolent communication, what you say and the words you choose come from your ability to respond (from a connection state), rather than react (from a protection state) to what is present. This is possible with awareness of your own physiological state (see Figure 11.1). Consider this: if you are in protection mode (fight, flight, freeze, or shutdown), rather than connection mode (rest, restoration, active engagement, play, and challenge), your words are more likely to come from habitual, defensive patterns and may be harmful or hurtful. Conversely, when you are self-aware and present, it is more likely your words will be reflective of what is present in the moment, intentional, thoughtful, and supportive of the students' experiences.

TIR PRINCIPLE: TRAUMA-INFORMED AND RESPONSIVE COMMUNICATION IS NONVIOLENT
Learn and practice the principles of nonviolent communication.

You are responsible for your own self-regulation as well as the impact of your words and actions on others. Before you take any of the steps listed below, take a moment and assess your state activation. If you are feeling activated and defensive (in protection mode), take some time to down-regulate your physiological and emotional systems. This might include waiting a day to calm down, sharing your experiences with a trusted other, practicing asana, doing grounding and breathwork, and practicing the PAUSE.

> **PRACTICING THE PAUSE**
> Any time, any place, and for any reason, you can always PAUSE. Pause = stop what you are doing, A = assess how you are and what you need, and USE = use your resources.

Nonviolent communication fuses ahimsa and satya. When communicating this way, you seek the truth within you and within those with whom you are communicating. Then, through the lens of ahimsa, you speak. You share your experience, what you observe, feel, and need. You listen, hearing what others observe, feel, and need. Together, you work toward understanding and meeting each other's needs. It is a beautiful, thoughtful, and powerful practice.

TIR PRACTICE: NONVIOLENT COMMUNICATION

Nonviolent communication is practiced using six basic steps (Lasater & Lasater, 2022; Rosenberg, 2012):

1. Make observations.
2. Name your feelings.
3. Express your needs.
4. Make a request.
5. Listen to and sense the needs of others (no matter how they express them).
6. Develop a plan that honors the feelings and needs of both, or all parties.

Step 1: Make Observations

When making observations, you seek to report facts, not beliefs, inferences, or judgments. Let's consider a common studio/organization issue. A favorite yoga teacher, John (he/him), consistently begins and ends yoga classes later than scheduled. The program manager needs to address this with John. The first step when speaking to John is to state the facts (Lasater & Lasater, 2022). According to Lasater and Lasater (2022), stating "You started the class late" is a judgment. Perhaps there is a back story and John was, in fact, late since the yoga class was scheduled to begin at 9:00 am. In this case, the observation would be: "You started the class at 9:10 am, ten minutes after the yoga class was scheduled to start." Judgments can result in a debate about what is true. John might think that starting class anywhere within a ten-minute window of when it started is fine. John might explain he knows the students in the class and about 80 percent of them show up late and would miss the introduction if he started at 9:00 am. Sandra (she/her), one of the yoga students, might believe that starting the class later than the scheduled time is late and not starting on time is disrespectful of people's time, rude, unprofessional, and inconsiderate. Sandra is upset that the class started late. In this case, John does not think he started the class late and Sandra thinks he did. She is also irritated and quite upset.

All of these are points of view and judgments around John beginning class at 9:10 am. Lasater and Lasater (2022) call judgment-filled statements pseudo facts or "a judgment masquerading as a fact" (p. 18). You might see how easy it is to argue about who is right here, losing the central issue of starting a class at the scheduled time. Emphasizing the importance of communicating in a clear, non-judgmental manner, Lasater and Lasater call the act of reporting observations and leaving out judgments and beliefs *spiritual speech*.

Judgments masquerading as facts:

- John started the class late.
- John is rude, unprofessional, and inconsiderate for starting the class late.
- By starting the class late, it is clear that John does not care about the students.

Observable facts:

- John started the yoga class that was scheduled to start at 9:00 am at 9:10 am.

Journal Prompt. Think of an experience or incident that occurred within the context of your yoga teaching. Something small you found a little irritating. If you can't think of one, you can create one to work with. Briefly, describe what occurred below. Write down any judgments masquerading as facts. Then review your description and write only the observable facts. Add any reflections on the ease or difficulty of this process.

Step 2: Name Your Feelings

Our feelings tell us about how we are doing in relation to ourselves, others, and what is important to us (our values, dreams, and reasons for being; Cook-Cottone, 2020). They arise throughout the unconscious and express themselves through body sensations. They can shift us from one state to another, such as feeling suddenly happy about some good news, moving from relaxed to alert, engaged, and joyful. Conversely, when we are threatened and feel angry, we may shift into a reactive fight or flight state (Cook-Cottone, 2020). Feelings are constantly arising, impermanent, and always changing (Lasater & Lasater, 2022). When practicing nonviolent communication, feelings are noticed, acknowledged, and shared. Being aware of and curious about what feelings come up and how you communicate those feelings can be very helpful in your quest to be a nonviolent communicator.

In nonviolent communication, feelings are understood as arising separate from what other people say and do and are unique to how you are experiencing the world (Lasater & Lasater, 2022). Other people's actions or words might trigger or stimulate your feelings, though your feelings remain unique to how you experience the world. When you share feelings using a nonviolent communication framework, the feeling used should describe your experience without involving others. Stick to what you can observe (inside and outside) and avoid the use of words that integrate assumptions and beliefs about others. You do not mix your expression of your feelings with analysis, judgment, or opinion (Lasater & Lasater, 2022).

Some basic feelings that can be useful within using nonviolent communication patterns:

Amazed	Angry	Annoyed	Anxious	Comfortable
Concerned	Confident	Confused	Disappointed	Discouraged
Distressed	Eager	Embarrassed	Frustrated	Fulfilled
Glad	Helpless	Hopeful	Hopeless	Impatient
Inspired	Intrigued	Irritated	Lonely	Moved
Nervous	Optimistic	Overwhelmed	Proud	Puzzled
Relieved	Reluctant	Sad	Surprised	Uncomfortable

The following statements are not aligned with nonviolent communication principles. Each include beliefs or assumptions about another person or expression of an analysis, judgment, or opinion.

- I feel like you are being difficult.
- I feel abandoned (hurt, betrayed, insulted).

- I feel like you don't care when class starts or your impact on students' practice.

The statements below are aligned with nonviolent communication principles. They stick to what you can observe in yourself, the world, and others. They do not include assumptions or beliefs.

- I feel sad.
- When I heard what you said, I felt sad (angry, anxious, frustrated, etc.).
- When you left earlier, I felt lonely and sad (angry, anxious, frustrated, etc.).
- When you start class after the scheduled time, I feel angry (Sandra).
- When you start class after the scheduled time, I feel concerned and confused (program manager).
- When you did x, y, z, I felt sad (angry, anxious, frustrated, etc.).

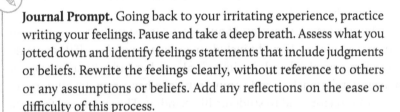

Journal Prompt. Going back to your irritating experience, practice writing your feelings. Pause and take a deep breath. Assess what you jotted down and identify feelings statements that include judgments or beliefs. Rewrite the feelings clearly, without reference to others or any assumptions or beliefs. Add any reflections on the ease or difficulty of this process.

Step 3: Express Your Needs

Nonviolent communication requires awareness and communication of needs. According to Rosenberg, the world-renowned nonviolent communication trainer, "needs can be thought of as the resources that life requires in order to sustain itself" (2012, p. 3). There are several types of needs. The list below is an example of several types of needs and some more specific needs in each category (Lasater & Lasater, 2022). This list is not inclusive of all needs. However, it can give you a good idea of some of the basic needs we share.

- Survival (e.g., air, water, food, clothing, shelter, safety, protection).
- Maintenance of the self/autonomy (e.g., to be seen, to be heard, identity, self-determination, sovereignty, freedom, integrity).

- Relationship and community (e.g., to be loved, affection, acceptance, understanding, touch, connection, emotional safety, trust, respect, belonging, participation).
- Thriving (e.g., play, intimacy, creative expression, recreation).
- Spirituality (e.g., peace, wholeness, meaning, purpose, connection with something bigger than ourselves).

Lasater and Lasater (2022) assert that needs are the way life expresses itself through our human form. When we are in touch with our needs, we are in touch with life itself. Accordingly, when our needs are not met, our fundamental humanness is denied (Lasater & Lasater, 2022).

It can be easy to get needs confused with strategies to meet needs. For example, "I need the yoga studio cleaned after each class." For the owner, this may meet needs like identity ("I keep a clean and organized studio") or survival ("If the studio is not clean, people will not come to class and I will not be able to make a living"). The strategy "I need a vacation" might reflect a drive for creativity and play or an escape from stress. It can be helpful to consider strategies used by yourself and others and what the underlying need might be.

John starting the yoga class at 9:10 am is likely stressful for the program manager whose needs might include maintenance of the self (keeping the yoga class organized and on time speaks to her integrity as a program manager), relationship, and community (she has a responsibility to the board of directors and to students like Sandra). The statement from the program manager might sound like this: "John, when I hear that you start the yoga class, which is scheduled at 9:00 am, at 9:10 am, I feel confused and concerned, because I need to honor and respect our relationships with our students and be in integrity."

Journal Prompt. Going back to your irritating experience, break it down into the three steps we have covered so far: (1) observable fact(s), (2) expression of feeling (without beliefs and judgments), and (3) expression of needs.

Step 4: Make a Request

When you make a request, you seek to meet your needs at that moment (Lasater & Lasater, 2022). Requests are (1) for the present moment and (2) doable (Lasater & Lasater, 2022). This is a good time to point out that nonviolent communication is about building and maintaining relationships, the connections between yourself and others. It is believed that through those connections, we can fulfill our own needs and the needs of others (Lasater & Lasater, 2022). The relationships are valued and central.

The general framework for a nonviolent communication looks like this (Lasater & Lasater, 2022, p. 29):

When I (hear, see, experience) _____,

I feel _____,

because I need _____.

Would you be willing to _____ (something now and doable)?

Using this framework, the statement from the program manager might sound like this: "John, when I hear you start the yoga class, which is scheduled at 9:00 am, at 9:10 am, I feel confused and concerned because I need to honor and respect our relationships with our students and do what I say I am going to do (be in integrity); would you be willing to talk to me for a few minutes about starting the class at the scheduled time?"

Journal Prompt. Going back to your irritating experience, add the final step to your statement. It might be helpful to write the whole statement together using the general framework for nonviolent communication. Remember, making the request must be something that is doable in the present moment.

Step 5: Listen to and Sense the Needs of Others (No Matter How They Express Them)

Since the goal of nonviolent communication is to meet the needs of everyone, mindfully listening and seeking to sense and understand the needs of others is critical to resolution. Rosenberg (2012) suggests the process of deeply listening and working to understand the other person's needs is the pathway to empathy. Your heartful and mindful listening practices are ideal here. If they are expressing a strategy, look for the need the strategy is designed to meet. As a practitioner of nonviolent communication, your practice will be to keep coming back to the inquiry "What needs is this person expressing here (no matter how they are expressing it)?"

In his meeting with the program manager, John explains he starts class at 9:10 am to include the students who have children to get to school and for whom transportation is unreliable. He explains that he does not want them to feel they are interrupting class when they enter after 9:00 am and he does not want the students practicing to feel interrupted. Although John expresses a lot of reasons for starting the class at 9:10 am, what needs do you think he is expressing here? The program manager might say, "John, it sounds like you are working hard to be inclusive and are worried about the students who can't get there on time, and the experience of those who do." Rather than being insubordinate, difficult, rude, and unprofessional, John appears to have a strong need for relationship and community. It will be helpful for the program manager and John to acknowledge these needs as they work toward a solution that will meet both the program manager's needs as well as John's.

Step 6: Develop a Plan that Honors the Feelings and Needs of Both, or All Parties

Together, the parties relevant to the issue at hand, aware of each other's concerns and needs, work to develop a plan honoring the experience and needs of all parties. During this step, continue to utilize mindful and heartfelt listening practices. Remember to focus on what can be done here and now and allow for solutions to evolve from your work. If you feel yourself pushing your agenda or feel a need to be right or in control, step back and practice your PAUSE. Then return to the six-step process.

There is so much more you can learn about nonviolent communication. Experiment with the steps above and take time to notice and journal about what you notice. Pay attention to how using this technique affects your relationships both within your yoga community and at home with your loved ones. If you'd like to learn more about nonviolent communication read *What We Say Matters: Practicing Nonviolent Communication* by Judith Hanson Lasater and Ike K. Lasater (revised edition, 2022).

TEACHER TRAINING DISCUSSION QUESTIONS

1. What are the steps for nonviolent communication?

2. Which steps do you feel are the most impactful in terms of shifting how you communicate during a conflict?

3. In what scenarios within your studio or organization do you see yourself using nonviolent communication?

CHAPTER 12

Content Warnings, Microaggressions, and Inclusive Language

sva-svâmi-åaktyoï svarûpopalabdhi-hetuï saäyogaï

Yoga Sutra II:23

The association of the Seer [the witness] with things seen [what is witnessed] is the cause of the realizing of [coming to know] the nature of things seen, and also of the realizing of [coming to know] the nature of the Seer.

Charles Johnston (1912)

Your skills in mindful, heartful listening and nonviolent communication will help you be more effective in your communication day to day and while experiencing conflict. Trauma-informed and responsive (TIR) yoga teachers are also well versed in how to deliver potentially triggering information, manage microaggressions, and use inclusive language. The goal is to be mindful of and effectively deliver or address content and information that may shift yoga students into a protection state (fight, flight, or shutdown). This chapter reviews each of the concepts and offers suggestions for most effective communication in these content areas. Consider Erica (she/her), a yoga teacher and full-time emergency medical technician (EMT), and Joelle (she/her), a yoga teacher, trainer, and nurse in a psychiatric unit at a local hospital.

> Erica is a yoga teacher who teaches yoga at a community center two evenings a week. Her full-time job is being an EMT. She frequently works in the midst of medical emergencies. Erica likes to vent about her EMT job

CONTENT WARNINGS, MICROAGGRESSIONS, AND INCLUSIVE LANGUAGE

and describe in detail the emergencies at which she has worked. It is not uncommon for her, before and after her yoga classes, to describe sexual assault victims, heart attacks, the state of neglected elderly individuals, and children in various states of injury. Some of the yoga students find her stories about work interesting. However, there are several students who find her stories upsetting and worry about the privacy of the patients she has treated. They wonder if she goes to work as an EMT and tells stories about the members of her yoga classes. Ultimately, it seems if you want to attend Erica's yoga classes, you will need to negotiate her venting and stories.

Joelle is a faculty member for a 200-hour yoga teacher training. She is trained and registered at the 500-hour level and teaches two yoga classes per week at a studio. She is a full-time job registered nurse at a local psychiatric center where patients are often suicidal, homicidal, and/or in need of medical stabilization. She rarely talks about this work in detail within the yoga studio. When someone asks her about her profession, she offers a general description: "I am a nurse over at City Hospital in a psychiatric unit." In the teacher training, Joelle teaches a section on stress, trauma, mental health, and wellness. When she does this, she lets the students know about the general topic area and gives them a sense of the specifics she will be covering. She does not disclose information about specific patients or events from work. Students tend to feel safe around Joelle. They know they can come to class early to lie or sit on their mats and even have a nice chat about the weather or yoga.

Journal Prompt. What are some key differences between Erica and Joelle? What might it feel like to be in Erica's class? Joelle's class? Which class might feel safer? Why?

After working through the chapter, come back and reflect on your answer here. Consider what advice or feedback you might give these teachers.

TIR PRACTICE: TRIGGER AND CONTENT WARNINGS

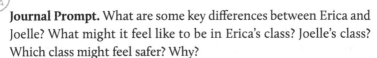

TIR communication includes mindfulness of your communication's content. For example, it can be helpful to avoid potentially triggering or violent words including phrases such as "beat a dead horse," "take a shot at it," "take a stab at it," "deadline," and "killing it" (American Psychological Association, 2022;

Gersen, 2021). TIR communication also means using techniques that let the listener know when you are going to say something potentially upsetting or triggering. During a typical yoga class or session, you likely won't need these types of warnings. This is more often an issue for workshops, trainings, and conversations in the yoga space.

To review terminology, a *trigger* is something that recalls a traumatic event to a person and may cause a re-experiencing or stress response. *Trigger warnings* are communications warning yoga students about forthcoming, potentially triggering content (Gersen, 2021). *Content warnings* (or *content notes*) are descriptions of the forthcoming content that offer students a chance to choose their level of exposure to the content. The debate surrounding whether or not to offer trigger or content warnings has been heated (Charles *et al.*, 2022). There is some research suggesting trigger and content warnings may either have no effect at all or increase anxiety for certain populations (Charles *et al.*, 2022). However, Bryce and colleagues (2022) counter that the evidence indicates that when trigger or content warnings are embedded as part of a broad, holistic, trauma-informed and responsive approach, they can be a valuable tool for reducing traumatization.

To effectively use content warnings or notes, embed them in the description of the content to be delivered, in your verbal overview before a workshop begins, and describe content before you deliver it. Be sure to flag content including potentially triggering themes such as violence, sexual abuse and assault, homicide, genocide, misogyny, segregation, slavery, racism, and/or domestic violence (Gersen, 2021). For example, "In this section of our discussion, we will be reviewing types of abuse." Aligned with this guidance, we provided a content warning in the Introduction of this book, informing you its content is centered around trauma with sections referring to trauma. We have also titled each chapter and included section introductions so you are aware of the forthcoming content and are empowered to make choices.

> **TIR PRINCIPLE:** USE CONTENT WARNINGS
> Using content warnings lets your students prepare for the content you will be delivering.

TIR PRACTICE: PRIVACY AND DISCRETION

Privacy is our right to make decisions about our private and personal matters. This includes personal information and the expectation of privacy within communication. *Discretion* means behaving or speaking in a manner that avoids causing offense or revealing private information. Respecting privacy and using discretion are two ways in which you can help your yoga students feel safer. Consider Erica. What message is she sending to her yoga students when she freely discusses the medical treatment of the patients she serves as an EMT? Is she respecting their right to make their own decisions about private and personal matters? What might you do differently?

> **TIR PRINCIPLE:** PRIVACY AND DISCRETION
> Honoring privacy and using discretion in what you share about others honors the trauma-informed values of personal agency and self-determination.

First, when considering what you might share about another individual with whom you work, ask yourself:

- "Is this my story to tell?"
- "Is this my information to share?"
- "Do I have permission to share this information?"

Ultimately, by honoring others' privacy, we are respecting their ability to control their personal information, their story. This aligns with the trauma-informed values of trustworthiness, self-determination, and empowerment. Second, consider the level of privacy available when you communicate about personal information with a student. Discussion about injuries, past trauma, fears, and body concerns can be best held within a one-on-one conversation (Karnes, 2023). For example, teachers often ask if anyone has any injuries, quite publicly, from the front of the room before the class begins. As a TIR teacher, you might consider a more private approach such as asking how they are doing and if they have any injuries during pre-class sign in or by checking in with students on their mats.

> **Journal Prompt.** Consider the settings and populations within and with whom you work. How might you address individual and communication privacy? How does the space within your work facilitate privacy in conversations? As a TIR teacher, what can you do to modify your approach to student privacy?

TIR PRACTICE: INCLUSIVE LANGUAGE
The recently adopted Yoga Alliance Code of Conduct requires yoga teachers to actively include all individuals (Yoga Alliance, 2020a). Inclusive means including everyone, especially those who have been historically excluded due to race, gender identity, size or shape, sexuality, mental health status, socioeconomic status, and/or ability. The American Psychological Association (2022) takes it one step further, defining inclusion as "an environment that offers affirmation, celebration, and appreciation of different approaches, styles, perspective, and experiences, thus allowing individuals to bring their whole selves (and identities) and to demonstrate their strengths and capacity" (p. 7). Inclusive practices include awareness of intersectionality. Intersectionality refers to the interconnected nature of social categorizations such as race, class, and gender that can create overlapping and interdependent systems of discrimination or disadvantage (Oxford English Dictionary, 2023). Kimberlé Crenshaw (2017) coined the term to speak to the dual discrimination experienced by African American women and to highlight how researchers tended to focus on their experience as either women or as African American. Crenshaw posits that our interacting identities converge to create how we are perceived, interpreted, and responded to by others—not only as a woman, or an African American, but as an African American woman. For more on intersectionality, see *On Intersectionality: Essential Writings* by Kimberlé Crenshaw (2017).

> **TIR PRINCIPLE: TRAUMA-INFORMED AND RESPONSIVE COMMUNICATION IS INCLUSIVE**
> Learn and practice using inclusive language.

Inclusive language, sometimes referred to as conscious language, is bias-free language that acknowledges and respects differences and treats all people with care (Ashwell *et al.*, 2023).

Inclusive language is inexorably tied to language itself. Language is collectively shared, influenced by social and political power dynamics, and has been used to justify racism, misogyny, genocide, and war. Language is socially constructed. It shifts and changes as our understanding shifts and changes. Language is also very personal. It is how we tell others who we are, what we love, and what is important to us. Here, we are seeking to provide you with guidance knowing that, as this text is published, things will likely be shifting and changing as they do when the public, political, and personal tensions shape the words we use.

Below, we seek to give you some initial guidance with the hope that you are inspired to continue your education in the areas of diversity, equity, and inclusion to further bolster your TIR teaching capacity. Surprisingly, there is little formal guidance on inclusive language within the yoga community. An internet search will yield many practitioner-based blogs, yet there is no published research and community-wide agreements within the yoga field from which to draw. In order to provide you with a combination of practice and professional guidance, we leaned on both practice-based blogs and guidance from the American Medical Association (2021), American Psychological Association (2022), and Yoga Alliance (2019, 2020a). We acknowledge the last three listed are institutions guilty of their own marginalizing, minoritizing histories and practices. We also acknowledge their recent guidance is their work to stop harmful practices and begin to communicate in ways that honor, empower, and include all people.

Consider the following specific guidance when communicating.

- Use person-first language. For example: "person who has experienced..." rather than "victim" or "survivor"; "person who uses a wheelchair" rather than "wheelchair bound"; "person living with a mental health condition" rather than "mentally ill"; "person with alcohol use disorder" rather than "alcoholic"; "person who was enslaved" rather than "slave"; "people whose incomes are below the federal poverty threshold" rather than "the poor," "low-class people," or "poor people"; and "formerly incarcerated" rather than "ex-con" or "felon" (AMA, 2021; American Psychological Association, 2022).
- For age; be specific: "persons 65 and older" rather than "the aged," "seniors," or "aging dependents" (American Psychological Association, 2022).
- For disability status, "person with a disability" rather than "special needs," "mentally or physically challenged," or "mentally retarded" (American Psychological Association, 2022).
- Refer to the race and ethnicity of others, as they identify: "students who identify as..." (e.g., Alaskan Native, Asian, Asian American, African American, American Arab, American Indian, Black, Hispanic, Indigenous Peoples, Latin(a/o), Latinx, Middle Eastern, Native Peoples, North African, White, multiracial, multiethnic) (AMA, 2021; American Psychological Association, 2022).
- Use the terms "people/persons of color," "communities of color," and

"people/communities with varying degrees of melanin." Do not use BIPOC (Black, Indigenous, and people of color). The term BIPOC was constructed to recognize that Black and Indigenous people are severely impacted by systemic racial injustices; however, it is considered by some to indicate a hierarchy among communities of color (APA, 2022).

- Use the term "historically marginalized/historically minoritized groups" to refer to racial and ethnic minority groups or individuals or underrepresented populations when referring to a disproportionately low number of individuals in a particular setting or community. The AMA (2021) encourages you to be specific: "Groups struggling against economic marginalization," "Communities that are underserved by/with limited access to (specific service/resource)."
- Use gender-neutral language (e.g., everyone, everybody, you, folks, folx, friends, persons, people, and chairperson) rather than "you guys" or "ladies and gentlemen" (APA, 2022). This includes not using gender-specific language cues like "Where your bra strap usually goes" (Karnes, 2023).
- Refer to the gender identity of others as they identify (e.g., cisgender, transgender, female, male, etc.; APA, 2022).
- Use a person's identified pronouns when you know them (e.g., he, she, him, her, his, hers, they, them, theirs), and when you do not know, ask or use they/them/theirs (APA, 2022).
- Avoid ableism and weightism in cues like "Just put your foot here," or "Simply come to standing" (Karnes, 2023).
- Avoid using words and phrases that can bring up historical and racial trauma or appropriate important spiritual and traditional terms and practices from other cultures.
- Avoid use of terms like "target," "tackle," and "combat" when referring to particular groups and communities (APA, 2022).

We encourage you to continue seeking training in these areas. We acknowledge this list of guidance, like all guidance related to inclusion and identities, can never be fully complete, and will be outdated as learning and practices evolve.

> **Journal Prompt.** Consider the settings and populations within and with whom you work. Where can you improve in your use of inclusive language? In what ways might some individuals not feel included in your yoga space or community? How can you shift that?

TIR PRACTICE: RESPONDING TO MICROAGGRESSIONS

Originally coined in the 1970s, the term *microaggressions* referred to subtle, nonverbal slights towards people of color (Costa *et al.*, 2023). The current, expanded definition of microaggressions is "commonly occurring, brief, verbal or nonverbal behavioral, and environmental indignities that communicate derogatory attitudes or notions toward a different *other*" (American Psychological Association, 2022, p. 5). Microaggression can include assumption of status (e.g., poverty, criminal, educational); ascription of intelligence based on race or other status; denial of racism, misogyny, weightism, anti-trans experiences; color blindness; ascribing to the myth of meritocracy (e.g., "Everyone can succeed if they work hard enough"); pathologizing cultural values and communication styles; treating others as second-class citizens; treating others as if they do not belong (e.g., "Where are you from?"; "Where were you born?"; or "You speak good English"); tokenism (i.e., asking an individual to speak for an entire group—"You are a person of color. Can you explain how this feels for people of color?"); and environmental microaggressions (e.g., all the buildings on a college campus are named after White males, or all of the faces on national currency are White men; Sue *et al.*, 2007).

> ## TIR PRINCIPLE: TRAUMA-INFORMED YOGA TEACHERS ADDRESS MICROAGGRESSIONS
> Be mindful of and address microaggressions as they occur.

Microaggressions accumulate over time and cause harm (American Psychological Association, 2022). A recent large meta-analysis of studies conducted on the effects of microaggressions found that they come at a cost, depleting personal protective and coping resources, and are associated with quantifiably and significantly reduced psychological wellbeing and physical health (Costa *et al.*, 2023).

As trauma-informed yoga teachers, we must work to identify and challenge our internal biases and oppressive ideologies with courage, self-regulation, and connection. In her book *Restorative Yoga for Ethnic and Race-Based Stress and Trauma* (2020), Gail Parker writes clearly and powerfully: "Unless we deal with our own discomfort regarding issues of race and ethnicity, and unless we learn the necessary tools to address emotional discomfort in a constructive, non-defensive, non-confrontational, non-avoidance way, opportunities for deeper understanding and connection are missed" (p. 47). Addressing microaggressions follows the principles of nonviolent communication (Souza, 2020). It is important to remember that microaggressions can be intentional or unintentional. It is possible the perpetrator may be unaware of their behavior and/or its impact (American Psychological Association, 2022). Coming from a nonviolent communication practice, there is no need to make assumptions about the underlying cause or agenda. The goal is to inform, teach, and call in rather than shame, embarrass, or call out (Souza, 2020). Souza (2020) describes this process as OTFD or Open The Front Door, or as the steps are called—Observe, Think, Feel, and Desire:

- **Observe.** State in clear language what you observed. As in nonviolent communication, state your observations without judgment. "I noticed an individual was asked to speak for an entire group" (Souza, 2020, p. 4).
- **Think.** Based on your interpretation and available evidence (what you observed), describe what you are thinking or can imagine others might be thinking or have experienced. "I think we need to resist this temptation because it is a lot, and might be harmful, to ask someone to speak for a whole community" (Souza, 2020, p. 4).
- **Feel.** Express how you feel about the situation. Here, as in nonviolent communication, take responsibility for open feelings using "I" statements. Specifically, name emotions without implying blame. "I feel uncomfortable with this request" (Souza, 2020, p. 4).
- **Desire.** State the specific, concrete action you would like to occur. This can include asking for the behavior to change or for more conversations about the microaggression. "I would like us to follow our group agreements and simply allow others to speak for themselves" (Souza et al., 2020, p. 4).

Ideally, this is done when the microaggression has occurred. However, if the setting does not seem conducive for effective exploration of the microaggression, engaging in a later, private conversation with the person who engaged in the microaggression can also be helpful.

> **Journal Prompt.** What is your experience with microaggressions? After reading through this section, do you think you may have perpetrated or been a receiver of a microaggression? How might the OTFD method be useful in this situation? Draft a possible OTFD statement.

TIR PRACTICE: MINDFUL USE OF SANSKRIT

Sanskrit is the language of yoga. Learning and using the Sanskrit and the English name of the pose provides education about the pose and honors the roots of yoga's South Asian heritage. This is only true if you do your research, study, and use Sanskrit correctly. The initial learning of Sanskrit words for poses can be challenging. This is where using good old-fashioned flashcards can be helpful. There are many resources available to support your learning.

Use caution and be informed. It is important to consider why you are using a Sanskrit word and what it is you are trying to convey. Author and Indian yoga practitioner Susanna Barkataki (2020) urges teachers to be mindful when using a language that is not their own. For example, she states her concerns about ending class using words like *namaste*. Her experience and usage of *namaste* is as a greeting *not* as a goodbye or as a convenient way to end a yoga class. It is also important to remember that context matters. In some cases and settings, students (and other organizational personnel) interpret use of Sanskrit as potentially religious or nonsecular. Even if this is not your intent or consistent with your beliefs about yoga and Sanskrit, some practitioners (and other organizational personnel) do not feel comfortable with its use. In settings such as schools, public hospitals, and treatment facilities, keeping your language simple, affirming, sparse, and inclusive is going to be most helpful.

Journal Prompt. Think of some ways that you might end your class other than using the word *namaste*. What words would signal that class has ended? What words would allow the experience of taking a yoga class to feel complete?

TIR PRACTICE: INDIGENOUS LAND ACKNOWLEDGMENT

Land acknowledgments are a traditional custom that date back many centuries (Native Knowledge 360°, 2023). Indigenous land acknowledgment is the effort to recognize the Indigenous past, present, and future of a particular location and to work toward understanding one's place within that relationship (American Psychological Association, 2022). These are often offered both in world and verbal statements. They are frequently delivered at community gatherings, events, concerts, and festivals (American Psychological Association, 2022). In order to provide an accurate land acknowledgment for your area, it can be helpful to reach out directly to local Indigenous communities and to Native Nations forcibly removed from your areas (Native Knowledge 360°, 2023). You can ask how they want to be recognized. You may consider offering a land acknowledgment at your yoga events as well as on your studio or organizational webpage. Note, it is important to offer acknowledgments as a regular practice, with reverence and deep respect and not as a performative action to check off of the dos and don'ts list for events.

Journal Prompt. Take a moment to reach out to your local Indigenous community(ies) and request the land acknowledgment that they would like you to use. Write this land acknowledgment in your journal. In which circumstances might you share this land acknowledgment?

Conclusion

Working through the communication chapters will help you create the communication foundation you need to step in front of a yoga class, workshop, or training, and support your students during informal conversations. Your communication choices support your creation and maintenance of a yoga space that is as intentional as your yoga practice in regard to how words are used, students are heard, problems are solved, and individuals are acknowledged and respected. From this grounded and thoughtful framework, the chapter of cueing, assisting, and invitational language will help you bring your words and actions directly and thoughtfully to your students' yoga mats.

TEACHER TRAINING DISCUSSION QUESTIONS

1. What is the difference between a trigger warning and a content warning?

2. What content warnings do you see as helpful in your yoga teaching and training?

3. How does privacy and discretion play a role in the words you use and stories you tell? How might your choices affect your students?

CONTENT WARNINGS, MICROAGGRESSIONS, AND INCLUSIVE LANGUAGE

4. In what ways does inclusive language create access to yoga spaces?
5. What are microaggressions and why are they harmful?
6. What can you do if you observe a microaggression?

CHAPTER 13

Trauma-Informed and Responsive Cueing and Assisting

saäskâra-sâkææât-karañât pûrva-jâti-jõânam

Yoga Sutra III:18

When the mind-impressions become visible [come to know the patterns of the mind], there comes an understanding of previous births [the patterns of the past].

Charles Johnston (1912)

Trauma-informed and responsive (TIR) cueing and assisting requires thoughtful consideration about the most helpful, supportive, and effective practices for each individual student. Due to the wide range of ways individuals have experienced and are at risk for trauma, cultural differences, differences related to gender norms, experience levels, and general comfort with touch and guidance, it is impossible to offer specific guidance in terms of "do exactly this and don't do exactly this." For example, for some, hands-on assists might be what is needed and wanted. For others, these same assists are experienced as a violation and triggering. Currently, there are no scientific research studies on the topic. Our guidance in this chapter comes from years of experience teaching yoga and leading yoga teacher trainings, and from the body of work in trauma-informed and trauma-sensitive yoga. This guidance offers multiple ways you can support self-determination and agency among your students.

The Importance of Active Facilitation of Choice

Trauma is about being overwhelmed, incapacitated, or having no choice (Cook-Cottone, 2023; Emerson, 2015; Emerson & Hopper, 2011; van der Kolk, 2014). Often in trauma, the body is immobilized in the face of danger (e.g., freeze or shutdown) or experiences reactive and unsuccessful attempts at fighting or fleeing (mobilization). All students, and especially students who have been through trauma or potentially traumatizing experiences, benefit from practice making choices and taking effective actions (Emerson, 2015; Emerson & Hopper, 2011). In yoga, effective work is done in the connection or ventral vagal states (i.e., rest, restoration, recovery, alert engagement, challenge, and growth). By always prioritizing choice, students are able to practice mobilizing (moving) and immobilizing (stilling) the body in connection to and in service of their bodies and souls. Movements, stillness, breathwork, use of prompts, and opting out are intentional, purposeful choices over which the yoga student has control, agency, and self-determination.

> **TIR PRINCIPLE:** EMPHASIZE INTENTIONAL, SELF-DETERMINED MOBILIZATION AND IMMOBILIZATION
>
> Yoga is the intentional, self-determined practice of mobilizing and immobilizing the body in service of the body and soul.

> **TIR PRACTICE:** ENCOURAGE CHOICE
>
> Emerson and Hopper (2011) and Emerson (2015) make a compelling case for yoga's role in allowing practitioners to practice making choices and taking effective action in the present moment. As Emerson puts it, in yoga, "choice making [is] an immediate body experience" (2015, p. 69). Yoga is an antithesis to a trauma experience, in which there are often no feasible or effective choices available. In yoga class, over and over again, asana after asana, practice after practice, your students have access to the practice of choice and effectiveness. As a TIR yoga teacher, your role is to support that practice in a way this is ultimately a self-determined, empowered experience for your students.

> **TIR PRINCIPLE:** OFFER PRACTICE MAKING CHOICES
>
> "Yoga offers a way to practice making small, manageable choices in relation to one's body" (Emerson & Hopper, 2011, p. 45).

It is important to note that the context of your teaching will determine some of the language choices you make as a teacher. Consider what offering choice looks like, feels like, or means in different physical and social locations. Consider for whom choice was not always a safe option. Identities and intersectionality related to race, ethnicity, sexual orientation, gender identity, socioeconomic status, age, ability, experience, privilege, and social standing all affect how much choice a student may feel they have regardless of your words. For example, teaching in a yoga studio where students voluntarily pay and come to your class is a very different context from teaching in a locked facility like a jail, prison, juvenile detention center, substance use recovery center, eating disorder clinic, or a mental health facility or hospital. Choice needs to be openly discussed as it relates specifically to your yoga class. For example, in a community studio, choice can include leaving the space (e.g., going to the bathroom to collect yourself), whereas locked facilities may not permit yoga students to leave the room during class. The reminders should be clear, explicit, modeled, and verbalized.

Journal Prompt. As you reflect on your teaching, it can be helpful to be in inquiry about the following:

- In what ways did my teaching, cueing, and supporting facilitate the agency, self-determination, and empowerment of the students in my class?
- Did my class offer clear points of choice that were explicitly verbalized or modeled?
- How did I respond to the student in my class who varied from my cueing and made other choices (both internally and externally)? Did I feel resentment? Did I wonder if they were being resistant to my teaching? Was I pleased they felt the freedom to choose? What subtle/overt signals do they receive that their choices were accepted, maybe even embraced?

TIR PRACTICE: DETAILED CLASS DESCRIPTIONS AND TEACHER BIOS

Class descriptions and teacher bios are some of the first places students begin making choices about their yoga experience. The descriptions on your webpage or other informative materials should explicitly and clearly detail the types of assisting offered in class while giving an overview of what a student might expect. Your teacher bio gives students a chance to get a sense of the teacher, their background, their teaching style, and their approach to cueing and assisting. From this first point of contact, the student has an opportunity to attune to their own body and have the information that they need to choose.

> Consider Eric (he/him), who is recovering from trauma. He decides, after reading the class description and the teacher bio, that he would, in fact, like to attend a class with physical assistance. Eric has been working on his Half Moon Pose and believes that a little guidance that includes physical touch would be helpful. Wonderful. The student has information and is making a choice.

> Consider also Jose (they/them), another student in recovery from trauma, who in no way wants anyone to touch them. They carefully check the class description and the teacher bios and select a class that promises no hands-on assists. Also wonderful—unless what they read is not true and they head into class only to be physically assisted as they are in Child's Pose. It is in this case that there is potential for harm. What happened here? Perhaps a new teacher took over the time slot? Maybe the teacher changed their philosophy on touch, and the webpage and their bio were not updated? What we do know is that Jose's ability to be self-determined and choose was undermined. As would have been helpful for Jose, both the class description and the teacher bios should be updated regularly and be closely tethered to exactly what happens in class.

Journal Prompt. Write a class description and bio that reflects your style and approach to assisting and touch. Are there any changes you have made from an existing bio or description? If so, what has changed and why?

TIR PRACTICE: MINDFUL USE OF YOUR VOICE

There is a popular saying often attributed to Maya Angelou: "People will forget what you said, people will forget what you did, but people will never forget how you made them feel." How you use your voice matters. The tone of your voice and the words you use are all filtered through your students' neuroceptive filter, which constantly scans for signs of safety or danger. Use your grounded, connected, authentic voice. Take your time. Let there be a spaciousness and ease around your words. To develop your voice, make an audio/video recording of your practice teaching so you can evaluate yourself. Take a deep breath, let it out, and watch and/or listen. Be kind and generous with yourself just as you would be to a trusted friend.

> **Journal Prompt.** How would you describe the tone and effect of your voice? How might your voice be experienced by a yoga student in general (e.g., grounded, authentic, falsely calm, anxiety-provoking)? What about a student who has experienced trauma?

TIR PRINCIPLE: OFFER EXPLICIT, ONGOING, INFORMED CONSENT
Consent must be clear, continuously given, and based on access to information.

TIR PRACTICE: USING CLARIFYING STATEMENTS EARLY IN THE CLASS

As a reminder, it can be helpful to make a general statement early in the class that your cues and guidance are suggestions, things the student can consider. Ultimately, they choose the intensity, depth, lightness, engagement, pace, and form. Amber Karnes (2023), a body-positive yoga teacher, encourages teachers to use language up front to communicate their efforts to create a yoga class that is low-pressure, free of judgment, non-competitive, and inclusive. Karnes explains her two main yoga class rules: *No Suffering* and *No Judgment*.

Karnes (2023) reminds students that they are the only ones who are in their bodies, know their bodies, and know the nature of the sensations they are feeling. For no suffering, she orients students to their bodies. She reminds them to discern between the sensations naturally inherent in yoga practices such as muscles stretching and working as opposed to shaking and trembling, and shifts in the heart and breath rate. Karnes encourages her students to notice signs to back off and try something else such as stabbing or throbbing pain, tingling, sharp pains at the joints, pressure-like sensations in the face or throat, and not being able to manage your breath. For no judgment, she works to create the conditions that would best support self-acceptance and choice. For example, she reminds students there are people in the room who have been practicing yoga for years as well as others who are just starting, and that their practice is their own.

> **Journal Prompt.** What might your introduction and welcoming statements sound like? What do you think is important for your students to remember from the start? Finding your own words, write a welcoming reminder statement to your students that reinforces choice and honoring their bodies and needs.

TIR PRACTICE: OFFER EXPLICIT, ONGOING, INFORMED CONSENT

First, *explicit consent* is the granting of permission for something to happen or an agreement to do something. Consent is something the students own. It is theirs to give and theirs not to give. At each point in your interactions with students (including your webpage and class descriptions), you are either empowering their ability to consent or removing their right to agency and self-determination.

Informed choice includes giving students enough information so they can engage in resource management, distress tolerance, and coping. Each student, depending on their health, injury status, the physical and emotional demands in their lives, and trauma history, has a limited amount of physiological, emotional, and energetic resources when they come to your class. Some people come to class with very little in their gas tank.

> Consider Sandra (she/her), who is working through years of domestic violence. She is a single mom of three children, works full-time, and often helps care for her sister's two children in her home after work. She has ongoing knee and hip pain on the right side from a fall down the stairs. While it is extraordinarily challenging for her, Sandra loves yoga. She often forgets she can make choices on behalf of her body without fear of retribution. The practice of making choices in itself is life-changing for Sandra. She likes to know what to expect throughout the class so she can manage her energy and emotional resources. It is very helpful for her when the yoga teacher lets her know the balance of challenging and restful poses and shares how long they

will be holding poses. It is also very helpful for Sandra to know when the next opportunity to rest and restore will occur. This way, she is able to assess her resources, her ability to manage the stress of holding a challenging pose, and her ability to cope with several repetitions of a pose that will place demands on her hip or knee. With an idea of the bigger picture of the overall class and upcoming challenges, she can pace herself and practice making effective choices for her body.

Some verbal cues that would be helpful for Sandra are:

- "A reminder that at any point in class you are welcome to take a restorative pose like Child's Pose..."
- "Today we will be working with Crescent Lunge Pose. We will begin on the floor warming up and working on flexibility. We will do a series of standing poses including lunges, and then move back to the floor and focus on our hip flexors and hamstrings."
- "I will be cueing four heart-opening poses for counts of five, ten, and 20. Options include Supported Bridge, Bridge, Camel, and Wheel."
- "You can remain here for another five breath cycles."
- "After these standing poses, we will be taking some time to restore in Forward Fold and *Malasana*."

Ongoing means that there are constant reminders of choice throughout the class, within the teaching of each pose, and within the general atmosphere. *Ongoing* does not mean a one-off statement in the beginning of class, or a plaque on the wall reminding students to make the best choices for their bodies and mind. Although statements and plaques are helpful, they are not sufficient. Ongoing reminders can include frequent reminders during class that students can choose a pose or version of a pose, where to place your mat, whether or not to use props, freedom to speak, be silent, or ask questions, and modeling of choice making.

- "As a reminder, all poses and versions of poses are encouraged."
- "All cues are optional."
- "All questions welcome."
- "Find a place for your mat that feels right for you."
- "Select the blocks, straps, and bolsters that you would like."
- "I invite you to meet your body wherever it is today."

> **TIR PRINCIPLE:** ESTABLISH THE FUNDAMENTAL CHOICE TO STOP
> To be trauma-informed and responsive, your yoga teaching must create access for your students to the fundamental choice to stop at any point.

TIR PRACTICE: OFFERING THE CHOICE TO STOP

Emerson and Hopper emphasize that the most fundamental choice is to stop at any point that feels right for the student. The message is "If you do not like the experience for any reason, you have control—you can stop" (2011, p. 45). A student is never stuck in a painful or uncomfortable position just because you cued it, as their yoga teacher. A student's choice should always come from their own sensations, feelings, and needs, not from the commands or expectations of the yoga teacher. Emerson and Hopper suggest once the fundamental choice to stop at any point is established, you, as the yoga teacher, can then offer additional choices.

> **TIR PRINCIPLE:** BE MINDFUL OF APPEASEMENT (OR FAWNING)
> Yoga students may engage in appeasement when they perceive a power differential, are seeking acceptance, and/or feel threatened.

Appeasement (or the Fawn Response)

There is a limited amount of research and some theory around appeasement or the fawn response to trauma (Scholte, 2023; Walker, 2013). The appeasement response is described as an attempt by an individual to minimize distress or danger by trying to please and appease the threatening person through submissive (i.e., yielding to force or threat), affiliative (i.e., forming social and emotional bonds), and inhibitive (i.e., holding back, or restraining) behaviors (Keltner *et al.*, 1997; Scholte, 2023). It is believed to be driven by autonomic states (recall the polyvagal theory) in which, under extreme stress, the nervous system engages the appeasement strategy in an attempt to co-regulate both the nervous system of the person at risk and the person causing the distress (Scholte, 2023). Walker (2013) is believed to have coined the term *fawn response* describing it as codependent behavior individuals use to prevent retaliation and/or harm in domestic abuse situations involving caregivers and partners. Ultimately, according to Scholte (2023), researchers suggest that the marginalized, appeasing person may feel less danger in the moment because of their actions, but still not feel truly safe given the potentially dangerous and/or threatening conditions.

Appeasement or fawning may have played a role in the non-consensual, abuse relationships that have occurred throughout the yoga community. In such cases, students may feel vulnerable, desire acceptance from a person in power, and have difficulty setting boundaries or are afraid to say "no" for fear of losing proximity to someone they consider their guru or mentor. The appeasement theory can help explain why a person in power may view an interaction as consensual, while the person who is socially situated with less power does not. This theory and research make clear, for you as a yoga teacher, in a social position of power, that it is possible any one of your students may be engaging in an appeasement response. You cannot use compliance with your requests and guidelines as a 100 percent assurance that the yoga students in your class are engaging in stress-free, willful consent. You must do everything you can to support agency and self-determination, and create an environment in which people can experiment, explore, and work on their relationship with choice.

A TIR yoga teacher will spend a lot of time asking themselves these questions:

- "Do my students truly believe they have a choice?"
- "What can I do to make choice truly accessible to all my students?"

Journal Prompt. What about you, your yoga students, and the social location of you and your students might impact a student's ability to feel that they have a choice? What can you do to increase their access to choice?

Trauma-Informed and Responsive Verbal Cueing

TIR cueing has four basic steps: inviting students into an asana or practice, orienting students toward interoception, offering options that are made based on interoceptive awareness, and encouraging choice (see Figure 13.1).

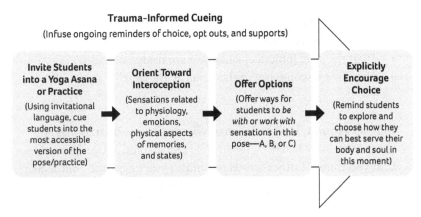

FIGURE 13.1 TRAUMA-INFORMED AND RESPONSIVE CUEING
(Informed by Cook-Cottone, 2015, 2023; Emerson, 2015; Emerson & Hopper, 2011)

TIR PRACTICE: INVITE STUDENTS INTO A YOGA ASANA OR PRACTICE

Choice is reinforced by how we cue (Emerson, 2015). This can be done through invitational language, by inviting students into yoga asanas or practices, rather than simply stating, calling, commanding, directing, or dictating a pose. Invitational language is a central TIR yoga teaching practice. Personal agency, self-determination, and practice making choices are highly important in a yoga class. What would be the benefit of forcing someone to move and breathe against their will? Spence (2021) states that making the willful choice to move our body and connect to our breath in some way should not be underestimated. It is how we remind our bodies and minds that we have choice, even if there have been times in our lives when we felt it or, quite literally, did not. The following are some examples of invitational language:

- "I invite you to..." (instead of "I want you to...").
- "If you want to, join me in raising your arms on your next inhale."
- "Would you like to try...?"
- "I invite you to sit in a comfortable position."
- "If you would like to, join me in linking your breath to your movement. Inhale, lift your arms. Exhale, lower them."
- "As you start to notice your breathing, feel free to have your eyes open or closed, whichever feels more comfortable to you."
- "Feel free to..."

- "Just for today, let's try…"
- "When you are ready…"
- "Exit the pose [practice] when you are ready."
- "Feel free to come out of the asana at any time."

Journal Prompt. How or in what ways do you use invitational language? For some teachers, it can feel cumbersome or overly wordy. Can you think of other words or phrases you might use so it feels more natural and concise? Write some ideas in your journal.

TIR PRACTICE: ORIENT STUDENTS TOWARD INTEROCEPTION

Once the student is in the pose or set up for a practice, orient their awareness toward their bodies and inner sensations (Cook-Cottone, 2023; Emerson, 2015). When practicing making choices to *be with* (e.g., notice and experience) and/or *work with* (e.g., taking effective actions), students need information from the body: "What is my body [knee, shoulder, back, legs, core, breath, or heart] feeling right now?" As a TIR yoga teacher, orienting the students toward their internal sensations (i.e., interoception), you are encouraging them to make informed choices on behalf of their own experience, their own bodies.

Use the word *your* to refer to part of the body ("your belly," "your foot," "your hands," rather than "the belly," "that foot," and "the hands"). Individuals who have experienced trauma and those who have grown up in a body-objectifying culture may have difficulty feeling a sense of connection with and ownership of their bodies (Cook-Cottone, 2020). Bringing everything together may look like this: "In Warrior 1, notice your front knee, the sensations in your calf, and thigh. Now consider, would you like to stay here and experience the pose as it is, soften the pose, or deepen into the pose? Notice your body as you choose." With caution against implying what is the right way to feel, you might, at times, share what you notice in your own body to model interoceptive awareness. For example, "In my body, I am noticing…" or "For me, it feels…" "What does it feel like for you in your body?" (Schmidt, 2020). Use words such as "Notice…" and "Bring your awareness to…" and "Consider the sensations…"

Refrain from telling students how they should feel (e.g., "This pose should feel really nice" or "You should feel a great stretch here"), even if they ask. You may notice some students will want your feedback as to whether they are "doing" the pose right and feeling the "right" sensation in a particular part of their body. Responding with "How does it feel to you?" or "What is your breath telling you?" or a variation of "If you are holding your breath, perhaps you are doing too much in the pose" are helpful ways to reframe poses to allow students to assess their own bodies' experiences rather than trying to copy you exactly. You are inviting your students to experience their own yoga journey.

> **TIR PRINCIPLE: OFFER OPTIONS**
> To make an informed, empowered choice, students need information about ways to accommodate, modify, or expand the pose.

TIR PRACTICE: OFFER OPTIONS AND ENCOURAGE CHOICE
To make an informed, empowered choice, students need information about ways to accommodate, modify, or expand poses (Emerson, 2015). Begin with the simplest, most accessible version of the pose, then add options. For example, in Crescent Lunge Pose:

> When you are ready, move into Crescent Lunge Pose. Step your right foot forward. Bend both knees, bringing your left knee to your mat. You might want to place a towel under your back knee to cushion. Bring your awareness to your knees and hips. Options include staying here and experiencing the pose as it is (*being with*) or *working with* the posture by (A) curling your back toes under and lifting through the back knee, (B) hands on your hips, or (C) hands reaching up toward the ceiling.

There are many ways to teach this pose and offer choices. Emerson (2015) guides his students to try options and, if they feel tolerable, stay with the option, and notice and feel (*be with* the posture). If the option does not feel tolerable, the student can begin to *work with* the posture: try one of the other options—when it's tolerable, stay, notice, and feel. Yoga teachers might also include use of blocks or bolsters. It is essential to begin at a supported version of the pose, encouraging interoception, and offering options to *be with* or *work with* the pose from there (Cook-Cottone, 2013; Emerson & Hopper, 2011).

- "Options include staying here and experience the pose as it is.

You might also _____ (option A), _____ (option B), or_____ (option C)."
- Sometimes you can add, "Or any other pose or action you'd like to take."
- "If it is painful, you can always stop" (Emerson & Hopper, 2011, p. 45).

As you frame options, speak in an empowering manner. For example, "You might like this version or you might expand the pose by x, y, or z." Your words should embrace and honor the most accessible version of any asana or practice and then offer choice—other ways to modify and expand. Students can feel embarrassed, weak, and engage in self-judgment if supports or modifications are framed as the easy way, the way for people who are stressed or struggling, or the way for people who are injured or traumatized. Your cueing can be received in this way: there is a good way (i.e., normalized or privileged way) and a bad way (i.e., the people who aren't capable of the good). A student who does not feel it is acceptable to take an accommodation may feel yoga is not for them, get injured, or feel too ashamed or embarrassed to come back to class. Using supportive and empowering language and speaking from the most accessible form of the pose first speaks to inclusion of all abilities, body types, experience levels, and injury statuses.

Table 13.1 Contrasting Supportive and Harmful Statements

Supportive and Empowering	Potentially Harmful
You might like this version or you might expand the pose by x, y, or z.	If you find this too hard or stressful, consider dropping your knee.
Chairs (blocks, bolsters, straps) can be a great support.	If you have limitations, you can use a chair.
Here are the options… Listen to where your body is today and choose the version that best aligns with what you need.	For those of you who can't do this pose, try…
In Down Dog, there are options to move to Table Pose, or walk out your feet, stretch your heels to the floor, or lift and stretch your left leg, opening the hip flexor and spreading your toes.	In Down Dog, just lift your left leg, open your hip, and spread your toes.
Explore which version of this pose feels right for your body right now. Let your sensations guide you.	The full expression of this pose is…
If you'd like to bring more heat into this pose, try…	The advanced or more difficult version of this pose is…

One Last Word on Trauma-Informed and Responsive Cueing—Frequency

It is important to match the frequency of your cueing to the needs of the students and the class. In some settings, such as a vinyasa studio with a core group of regulars with whom you are well acquainted with knowledge of personal histories and injuries, less frequent reminders of choice may be appropriate and/or wanted. In other settings, such as a recovery center for domestic violence or other relational trauma, frequent reminders (perhaps at each pose) might be what is needed for students to begin practicing choice making. Often it is not so clear. For example, it might be the studio-based vinyasa class that needs reminders as the students compete, judge themselves, and regularly work themselves to injury and distress. Meanwhile, the students at the domestic violence shelter may need fewer reminders since they are consistently working on choice and agency, and your yoga class is another place to engage in this internally motivated practice. There are several factors to consider when assessing the frequency of TIR cues needed in each yoga session:

- any known trauma history
- tendencies to push too hard, compete, or work to injury
- yoga experience (in general, with you, with the studio)
- interactions among you, your identity and social location, and the students' identities and intersectionality—for example, age, gender identity, race, ethnicity, socioeconomic status, abilities
- setting (prison, studio, rehab center)
- power and group dynamics
- overall setting culture (permissive, competitive, restrictive)
- most importantly, what you observe.

Additionally, while each factor is useful and important information, in some settings you may never know the answers. In such situations, your observations are even more important.

Journal Prompt. Consider the settings and populations within and with whom you work. Explain the factors that are important for you to consider when determining how frequently you should offer TIR cues (as described above).

Hands-on Assisting—To Do or Not to Do?

Hands-on assisting (i.e., guiding, facilitating, and/or deepening students' postures and practices through hands-on touch) is part of the yoga tradition. Touch, in general, cannot be framed as good or bad. In some cases, it is exactly the right thing, and in other cases, it can do harm. Judith Hanson Lasater, in her book *Teaching Yoga with Intention*, illustrated the many ways we touch others, describing it this way:

> Touch is a sacred act... We touch people with our hands, but we also touch people with our smiles, our teachings, our words, and our actions. All day long we are "touching" the people around us by the choices we make in word and deed. (Lasater, 2021, p. 45)

TIR PRACTICE: CAREFULLY CONSIDER TOUCH AND HANDS-ON ASSISTS

David Emerson, in his book *Trauma-Sensitive Yoga in Therapy: Bringing the Body into Treatment*, explicitly states: "In TSY [trauma-sensitive yoga], there are *no* physical assists. The facilitator will never place his or her hands on a client in the context of TSY" (2015, p. 74; emphasis in original). Recall that his work is with individuals who have experienced trauma and are in treatment. He described the scenario guiding him to this decision. He reported initially that he felt individuals who have been through trauma would benefit from safe touch. Through client feedback, Emerson found no matter how invitational the language, touch was experienced as an indication the client was doing something wrong or was being asked to do something with their bodies they didn't want to do, and/or the touch triggered dissociation. Emerson was deeply concerned that the experiences clients were having as a result of touch were not aligned with the words the yoga teachers were using. It is a classic example of intention versus impact. Within the context of their work with their clients, touch was not going to work.

In other cases, the experience is different. Consider individuals who have a history of sexual abuse. Gentle assists (following explicit, informed consent) in yoga class can be an opportunity to experience non-sexual, supportive touch. For some students whom you assist in yoga class, it can be a transformational experience to be touched intentionally in a way that is not related to a sexual advance or physical punishment. Hands-on assists can offer some yoga students a new perspective on experiences of human contact—it could be supportive, non-threatening, within their control and choice, and safe. Judith Hanson Lasater (2021) describes other instances in which touch might be helpful, including when a student's alignment might cause injury, when the assist might enhance the pose for a student, to remind a student to soften or do less in a pose, and/or to touch a student while they are volunteering to enhance the modeling of the alignment of a pose for a class (Lasater, 2021).

For certain, this is an area in need of research to facilitate better understanding of the impact of touch. It is not difficult to provide many examples of the benefits as well as those that reflect the risks inherent in hands-on assisting and touch. Ultimately, the safest approach is to not do hands-on assists or touch your students at all. However, this approach does not leave space for the potentially helpful role touch can play in yoga and being. For now, given the body of evidence from which we can draw, it will be important for you to carefully and intentionally develop your policy around touch, secure training, and engage in ongoing self-study.

Consider the following as you develop your approach to touch in your teaching:

- Bear in mind Judith Hanson Lasater's motto about touch: "When in doubt, don't" (2021, p. 64).
- Use class description and teacher bios to describe the touch and assisting policy for the class and the philosophy of the teacher.
- Before using touch, try verbal cues, demonstrating the pose, asking an assistant to demonstrate the pose, and using hand gestures to indicate where a body part might be moved (e.g., point to a place on the mat and state: "If you'd like, try moving your foot here") (Lasater, 2021).
- To touch or physically assist (hands-on assist) a student, you must ethically secure explicit and informed consent from the student (Yoga Alliance, 2019, 2020a, 2020b). This means they clearly and explicitly inform you that they do want to be given hands-on assistance (Yoga Alliance, 2020a).
- Explicit, informed consent can be provided verbally, in writing (as part of the waiver and liability process), by a clear gesture (e.g., a private thumbs-up in Child's Pose), or via a consent indicator (e.g., a consent card, chips; Yoga Alliance, 2020a).
- Consider that explicit, informed consent may be for a specific teacher, teaching assistant, or group of teachers, and this should be clarified as part of the informed consent process (Yoga Alliance, 2020a).
- Use consent cards, chips, or another signal that can be used for

consent, and changed as the student shifts their consent (e.g., "I no longer want to receive assists in this class").
- Silence, no response, and/or lack of resistance does not equal consent (Yoga Alliance, 2020a).
- Consent given at any one point in time does not equal ongoing consent, future permission, or allowance of physical adjustments (or contact of any type) in the future (Yoga Alliance, 2020a).
- The consent process should be confidential. For example, all students have consent cards and chips, so it is less obvious who is opting in or out. This reduces social pressures to appease or be agreeable.
- Encourage students to check in with their bodies, do their own self-reflection throughout the class, and shift their consent in accordance with what they notice (Yoga Alliance, 2019). This may look like deciding to try assists after the first part of class, or deciding to opt out of assists for *Savasana*.
- Know why you are touching students. Avoiding fixing or correcting. Use touch to "inform the conversation the student is having with their body in the pose at this moment" (Lasater, 2021, p. 50).
- Never touch students in or near sensitive areas such as areas near genitals, breasts, under arms, inner thighs, and undersides of feet (Lasater, 2021).
- Be clear that you know your intention, why you are engaging in touch, and how you will touch the students (Lasater, 2021).
- Move slowly, use just enough pressure, and use the least contact necessary (Lasater, 2021).
- Consider medical recommendations for touch in regard to disease transmission during times such as the COVID-19 pandemic. Use a disinfecting cloth or lotions between assists to decrease the chance of transmitting bacteria or viruses.

A Case Study: Touch, Consent, and Confusion

For years, I (JS) have been steadfast in my recommendation to not touch students during a yoga class. We need to use our words and our tone of voice to instruct. However, I am also cognizant of the deep healing potential of therapeutic touch. It has to be by consent every single time. At the same time, when you do have consent, you need to be very cautious and intentional about touch. The following story is an example of how even with the best of intentions, things can go wrong.

I was invited to teach a regular yoga class at a youth detention center. I said yes, on the condition that all the staff experience a yoga class and some basic training on what yoga offers us. This approach, training the staff first, worked well to blaze the path for successful programming. There was always a staff person present in each youth class. Sometimes a staff person would simply take the class with the youth, sometimes they would observe, and on occasion they would even assist in teaching the class.

During a class one day, Tony (he/him), a yoga teacher in training, was with me. He had asked to assist and was genuinely curious about youth yoga in a detention center. I introduced my assistant and explained his role and why he was there, then mostly forgot he was in the room. The class was moving along nicely and there wasn't anything in particular for Tony to do. Then we got to *Savasana*, or Resting Pose as we called it. One of the youth, Ronald (he/him), who had taken the class before, requested the eye pillows and the "assist" I had given in a previous class.

I asked if I could demonstrate the "assist" on him so everyone knew what he was talking about. He agreed. I demonstrated on Ronald, and he gave everyone the two thumbs-up when I asked if he recommended the "assist." It included squatting near his head and using my two thumbs to sweep across the forehead, then placing light pressure on both shoulders with my hands. Then I would move around to Ronald's feet and gently lift them off the floor and give them a slight swing from side to side. I explained what I was doing as I was doing it. After Ronald's two thumbs-up, I said, if you want this "assist," place your hands on the floor. If you don't want the "assist," place your hands on your chest. Someone asked me to repeat the options again and I did.

I was working my way around the circle and it was going very well, when Tony started doing the "assist" too. He didn't get far because the next person he went to—even though he was giving the sign for "yes, I want an assist"—was Derrick (he/him). Derrick sat bolt upright and said loudly, "Get your f#%#ing hands off of me." It was a rattling moment. There were so many things I wish I had done differently before and during this reaction. What I did do was own the mistake. I knelt beside Derrick and told him I was very sorry for not explaining Tony's offer to help. I asked him if he still wanted an "assist" from me. I was so relieved that he did. Tony had the sense to step back. We debriefed later. Derrick was actually able to reset and enjoy the "assist" and the rest time—it was a real credit to the resiliency of his nervous system. The yoga was working. I did not make the same mistake again.

Journal Prompt. Reading about Joanne's (JS's) experience, what stands out for you? Consider the importance of touch, safe touch, and the role it might play. What would you have done differently? Why?

Conclusion

I (CCC) wish this chapter could be more absolute, direct, and exact. However, if it was, we would lose the essence of yoga—attuned, compassionate connection, which does not and cannot be forced to look any particular way. Trauma-informed and responsive cueing and assisting is a yoga student-centered practice. Foremost is the experience, agency, self-determination, growth, and healing of the student. Anything functioning as a barrier between a student and their relationship with their yoga practice, whether it be a verbal or hands-on assist, does harm. This work of being a TIR yoga teacher is ongoing and filled with years of refining your personal approach. Perhaps by the time we write the next edition of this book, my research team, or another, will have explored concepts like hands-on assisting in depth and we will be able to give research-informed guidance. For now, we work with the case studies, theory, and the centuries of guidance that we have and do our best to support our students and their yoga practice.

TEACHER TRAINING DISCUSSION QUESTIONS

1. Why is intentional, self-determined mobilization and immobilization important for yoga students within the context of trauma? (Think polyvagal theory as you consider your response.)

2. Discuss why *choice* is so important within a TIR yoga class.

3. Describe what explicitly, ongoing, informed consent meant to you. Give an example from a yoga class.

4. What is appeasement, or the fawn response, and why is it important for a TIR teacher to be mindful of the process?

5. Describe the step-by-step process of trauma-informed cueing.

6. Detail the issues involved in developing a personal and/or studio/organizational policy on touch.

PART IV

TRAUMA-INFORMED AND RESPONSIVE YOGA TEACHING PRACTICES

PART IV

TRAUMA-INFORMED AND RESPONSIVE YOGA TEACHING PRACTICES

CHAPTER 14

Teaching Self-Awareness and Attunement—Being With and Working With

santoæâd anuttamaï sukha-lâbhaï

Yoga Sutra II:42

From acceptance, the [practitioner] gains happiness supreme.

Charles Johnston (1912)

Yoga practice is the opportunity to develop and nurture our relationships with our bodies and physiological states, emotions, and thoughts (see Figure 14.1). Trauma-informed and responsive (TIR) yoga teaching centers on cueing students to notice, truly see, and listen to what their nervous systems are telling them while responding in an attuned and connected manner in service of their growth and wellbeing. Teaching and guiding students in *being with* and *working with* skills empowers your students, supporting their capacity for agency, self-determination, and self-regulation.

It is a misnomer that TIR yoga teaching is, uniformly, a series of calming postures and practices. Although it is true that a nervous system that has experienced trauma often needs to be calmed and soothed, what matters more is the ability of the human being living with that nervous system to be attuned and responsive to the present. This involves noticing the activation, deactivation, disintegration, overwhelm, and potential shutdown of their nervous system. Then, to attune to what is noticed, pause and respond by engaging in practices the nervous system needs to remain in connection, intention, and effectiveness. To teach this means using what we learned about trauma, the polyvagal theory, and associated sensations, emotions, and thoughts. It means using this knowledge to honor agency, choice, and self-determination while facilitating self-awareness, attunement, and integration of the mind.

The cueing we reviewed in Chapter 13 pointed to guiding students to intentionally *be with* and *work with* what is present. This chapter focuses on awareness and attunement with an emphasis on the pause before we take action: the powerful role of *being with* what is, before *working with* what is. It serves as a bridge to Chapters 15, 16, and 17 which describes *work with* practices that help shift the nervous system from one level of activation to another. Ultimately, it is our hope that through their yoga practice, students develop the awareness and skills needed to effectively choose how to be with or work with what is present for them in yoga class and in their lives.

The Yoga Mat as a Sanctuary and Learning Space

The yoga mat, a small rectangle of rubber or fabric under our bodies as we practice, is both a sanctuary and a learning space (Harris, 2021). It is a place upon which we can be free of our commitments, struggles, and challenges and focus on our connection to our own hearts. It is a space where we can try new things, fall, fail, sweat, and cry. We can learn to listen to our bodies and see what happens when we don't. As TIR yoga teachers, our work is, at least, to not get in the way of that process and, at best, to support, model, and guide in a manner that lets students find their own way. Before you teach, seeing students roll out their mats, remember this.

Observation

Part of your job is to observe your students, so keep your eyes open. Be attentive to the whole class. As you observe your students during the class, pay attention to signs of tension they may be exhibiting. If you observe tension in a student's face as they move, a gentle reminder to soften the jaw or relax the face will help them bring awareness to this tension. If you have trouble seeing tension in another's body, it does get easier over time. A fun practice is to sit in front of a mirror and tense different body parts, just to get used to seeing what it looks like. Trust that your students are the experts on themselves and their own experience. Over time, with your support and guidance, your students will develop a level of awareness regarding which practices may best suit them in a particular movement.

TIR PRACTICE: INTENTIONALLY BEING WITH WHAT IS THERE

As a teacher, you will need to balance the predetermined structure of your yoga class with the attunement needed to respond to your students. At any given time, a yoga student is feeling a whole host of sensations, emotions, and thoughts—some of them having more to do with memories and habitual reactions than with the present moment. As shown in Figure 14.1, engaging in a yoga posture or practice creates the opportunity to rework relationships with sensations, emotions, and thoughts and to orient toward and experience what is there (*be with*).

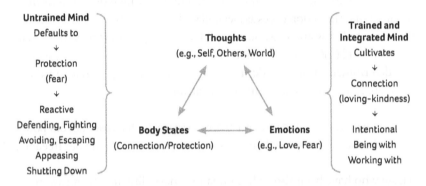

FIGURE 14.1 THE NATURE OF RELATIONSHIPS WITH BODY, EMOTIONS, AND THOUGHTS

In our culture, there is a tendency to move immediately to fixing, or *working with*, what is there. This shift to action takes away a powerful opportunity to be with what is present, right here, right now, and to learn and grow from what is experienced. The *be with* and *work with* model presented in Cook-Cottone (2020, 2023) honors the PAUSE *being with* can offer, while still utilizing the powerful tools available for *working with* what is present. *Being with* offers students an opportunity to do what Amy Weintraub (2012) calls *meeting the mood*. To do this, it is important to take time and be with the nervous system exactly where it is. Rather than try to shift things radically, you engage in a practice aligned with what is present and slowly work your way in the desired direction—to calm, energize, or balance.

> **TIR PRINCIPLE:** BEING WITH CAN BE TRANSFORMATIONAL
> Being with sensations in the present moment can be a transformational experience.

Desikachar (1995) points out that we achieve a state of yoga by what we do and don't do. *Being with* can be transformational. There is a lot to be experienced, known, understood, and discerned while in a yoga posture or practice. It is by being with sensations that we can come to understand their association with the present moment, our emotions, memories, our feelings of safety, and the action urges associated with the sensations. This is how we can come to know and trust ourselves. There is a quote, often attributed to Viktor Frankl (1962), that underscores what we can access—choice, agency, self-determination, and freedom—when we (and our yoga students) are able to create space while experiencing sensations:

> Between stimulus and response there is a space. In that space lies our power to choose our response. In our response lies our growth and our freedom.

Those who have been through trauma may have difficulty being aware of, noticing, and being with sensations. Sometimes it is very triggering. Sometimes it can be hard to feel anything at all. In TIR yoga, all of these experiences are welcome. If needed, use the tools in Chapter 3 to take a pause and support your students if they become activated or overwhelmed. You can also use the tools in Chapter 10 (mindful and heartful listening) to support students seeking to share their experiences. At any time, you can practice the PAUSE.

> **PRACTICING THE PAUSE**
> Any time, any place, and for any reason, you can always PAUSE. Pause = stop what you are doing, A = assess how you are and what you need, and USE = use your resources.

TIR PRACTICE: BEING WITH THE QUALITIES OF SENSATIONS

It is important to take time to be with sensations, noticing their qualities, and working to expand your window of tolerance—or the ability to be with all kinds and intensities of sensations without reacting or getting stressed. By pausing and *being with*, students can more intentionally choose their next move—stay and experience more or try something to soothe, calm, activate, stimulate, balance, or integrate in a way aligned with what will serve their wellbeing and growth.

Like meditation, a yoga posture (or asana) is a wonderful opportunity to pause and explore the various qualities of the sensations present.

- What is the sensation telling you about this pose, this moment, your body?
- What does it feel like? Soft, heavy, sharp, burning, empowering, expanding, contracting, and/or painful?
- Where is the sensation in the body? A specific spot? The whole body? A pressure point? A belly ache that feels like sadness?
- Is it comfortable, neutral, and/or uncomfortable?
- Do you feel a strong action urge with the sensation? Do you want to get away from it? Move? Connect? Keep it around? Avoid it?
- If the sensation could talk, what would it want? What would it say?
- Do you notice the sensations arising, peaking, and passing? What is that like?
- What is it like to simply notice and feel a sensation, or let it pass?
- If you don't feel anything, what does that feel like?

Journal Prompt. The next time you practice, take time to be with a few of the sensations you experience. Ask these questions. Write in your journal what you noticed and/or learned.

TIR PRACTICE: BREATHING—A POWERFUL BEING-WITH PRACTICE

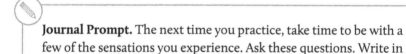

How you breathe matters. Stephen Porges (2017) gave us a new understanding of the breath as the most direct access to the nervous system. Most people without training in breathwork take breath for granted and fail to understand the connection between breath and wellbeing. A yoga class is a perfect place to introduce the benefits of breathing and its practice in a way that supports your students' wellbeing physically, mentally, or spiritually. Generally speaking, if you are not integrating awareness of breath, you are not doing yoga. Despite the breath being central to the practice of yoga, many students leave a yoga class never hearing "Bring your awareness to your breath," or even any reference or instruction as to how to breathe or link breath to your movement. As a TIR yoga teacher, set a firm intention to highlight the breath in each and every class you teach. Look around and observe how your students are breathing. Encourage: "Notice your breath?" Next: "Notice how you are breathing, whether through the nose or the mouth." Then, teach skillful breathwork.

> **TIR PRINCIPLE:** HIGHLIGHT BREATH IN EACH AND EVERY CLASS
> Set a firm intention to highlight the breath in each and every yoga class you teach.

Breathing in ways other than one's typical patterns of breathing is a new experience. It can be triggering for some and evoke feelings of self-consciousness in others. Set up practices so students feel grounded and well supported. Let them know they can opt out for any reason. Invite them to experiment. Offer choices to close or soften their eyes. It is good practice to remind your class if they feel dizzy or nauseated to take a PAUSE. You are encouraging students to listen to the wisdom of their own body and the magic of their own breath (and in doing so they are caring for themselves in that moment).

> **Journal Prompt.** What are you noticing about your breathing as you learn to teach asana? Has there been a time when you felt self-conscious about trying a new breath practice? What was that like for you?

TIR PRACTICE: BEING WITH—THE EIGHT LIMBS, GROUNDING, AND BREATHING

It is true that extensive and/or advanced breathwork can be dysregulating and/or triggering depending on the person and context. That said, it is important to teach breathwork within the context of all eight limbs of yoga, especially asana. In a meta-analysis of yoga for PTSD, Holger Cramer and colleagues (2018) found yoga had small, positive effects on posttraumatic symptoms, but for *not* breathing-only yoga interventions. This analysis of available research suggests that, to be effective, it is helpful to integrate breathwork with the other important aspects of yoga, especially asana.

Consider that the order of the eight limbs of yoga is hierarchical. They build on one another. You have learned or will learn the eight limbs of yoga in your training. As a review, the yamas (practices for relating with the world), niyamas (practices for relating with ourselves), and asana (physical postures) come before pranayama (energy and breathwork). When we honor the hierarchical nature of yoga, breathwork is practiced on a foundation of concepts such as nonviolence (ahimsa), satya (truth), tapas (self-discipline), and svadhyaya (self-study). It is also practiced with a physically grounded body in postures such as *Tadasana* (Mountain Pose), *Balasana* (Child's Pose), and *Sukhasana* (Easy Pose). By working through the limbs toward pranayama, the body can be stable and supported as it breathes.

> **TIR PRINCIPLE:** DEVELOP SKILLS TO BE WITH EMOTIONS
>
> Help students develop skills for being with their emotions and associated sensations.

TIR PRACTICE: BEING WITH—RIDING THE WAVE OF A SENSATION ACTION URGE

Sensations are often accompanied by an action urge. This can be especially true if you are experiencing a strong emotion or are in a protection state (e.g., fight/flight). Action urges come with their own set of sensations, arising and passing much like sensations do. They are distinct from other sensations, coming in the form of an urge, a compelling feeling you need to do something. Part of expanding the window of tolerance and working in the growth zone is to take time and be with action urges as they arise and pass without acting on them. Riding the wave is like surfing. You don't try to fight, resist, or control the wave. You simply breathe and ride it out. This does not mean enduring pain or ignoring your intuition. It is about pausing and being with the urge long enough to see it arise and pass. There might be something interesting driving it, and you may or may not want to act on it from a place of real choice rather than reaction. For example, I (CCC) sometimes get an urge to fidget in *Savasana* when I am heading into a busy or stressful day. However, if I let it be, rise and pass, I get to see it for what it is: my anxiety about the day. I remind myself that, right now, I can rest and let my yoga practice settle into my body. This is helpful in yoga class. It is also helpful in my life as I continue to explore my use of busy-ness as a coping strategy.

> **Journal Prompt.** Your next yoga practice, notice when you are feeling an action urge. Making sure this is not about safety or injury, experiment with what happens if you simply be with the urge. What did you notice?

TIR PRACTICE: BEING WITH—HAND OVER HEART

The hand-over-heart practice is a relatively simple practice to support being with emotions and the sensations associated with emotions. You can practice standing, sitting, or lying down. If you (or a student) are feeling as though you are becoming activated, upset, feeling a big feeling, or struggling with an uncomfortable sensation, place a hand over your heart and breathe gently. You are not trying to fix anything; this is a *be with* technique. You might say something validating to yourself such as "What I am noticing and feeling is difficult." It can be even more comforting to press your hand into your chest gently while making small circles on your heart area. You (or your student) can engage in this practice for as long as you like. It can be helpful to note your self-regulation rating before and after this practice.

TIR PRACTICE: BEING WITH—PENDULATION

The pendulation practice is a wonderful resource for coping with difficult emotions, memory-based sensations, and action urges as they show up (Cook-Cottone, 2023; Levine, 2010). In pendulation, you practice being with difficult sensations by moving your awareness to a spot in your body that feels neutral (see Figure 14.2). By moving your awareness back and forth, the activating or uncomfortable sensation is given more context. It reminds you, and your nervous system, that there are parts of you feeling just fine right now. Below is a script for guiding students through pendulation.

Sit down or lie down in a way that feels grounded and well supported. Bring your awareness to your body and where you are feeling uncomfortable sensations the strongest. Notice the intensity, size, and where the boundaries are—where does it end? Where are its edges? Breathe gently and intentionally and spend about four breath cycles (inhale, exhale four times) noticing this area of your body.

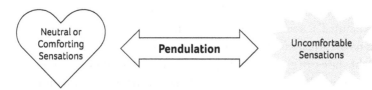

FIGURE 14.2: PENDULATION

Now, scan your body and find a spot that feels neutral or comfortable (a toe, your hands, the crown of your head). If you don't think you have a neutral or comfortable spot, consider the area right outside of your body—one inch around your body, six inches, a foot, or even two feet around your body. Bring your awareness to your neutral space wherever it is. Breathe there for about four breath cycles noticing your neutral place.

Now, move back to the place where you felt the uncomfortable sensations. Breathe there for about four breath cycles. Pendulate back to the neutral space. Breathe there for about four breath cycles. Do this a few times, pendulating from one spot to the other.

Last, bring your awareness to both the place where you felt the sensation the strongest and the neutral or comfortable place. Breathe while you hold this dual awareness of both places for about four breath cycles.

Journal Prompt. Try practicing pendulation on your own. What did you notice? Describe the place where you felt the uncomfortable sensation the strongest, the neutral place, the process of pendulating, and the process of holding both places within your awareness.

TIR PRINCIPLE: TRAUMA AND STATE ACTIVATION CAN SHAPE THOUGHTS
Invite students to notice, name, and reorient their thinking patterns.

TIR PRACTICE: BEING WITH—NOTICING, NAMING, AND REORIENTING THOUGHTS

Recall the chapters on trauma symptoms and indicators of your current state (connection and protection). Trauma symptoms include trauma-based cognitions (e.g., "I am not safe," "I am not worthy of protection," and "I am overwhelmed"). Similarly, the protection states of fight or flight and shutdown have corresponding cognitions. For example, cognitions aligned with the fight state can sound like "I hate this." The flight state can sound like "I am out of here." Shutdown can sound like "I can't ever do anything right." To help you recognize them, there are a few qualities to watch for. If we are not mindful, these thoughts can coalesce into stories or narratives we tell ourselves. It can be helpful to see them for what they are and reorient ourselves to the present moment. Note, if you or a student are struggling with persistent, ruminative thoughts (i.e., thinking the same negative thoughts over and over), consider reaching out to seek support of a mental health professional as this can be a symptom of anxiety, depression, and/or PTSD.

Trauma and protection state thoughts tend to be:

- personal—"I can't do anything right"
- global—"Everything is always bad" and "I will never be safe"
- certain—"This is 100 percent the way it is"
- permanent—"Nothing will ever change"
- negative—"This is the worst."

They tend not to take into account:

- the common human experience—"We all fail sometimes" and "Being human can be difficult"
- probability and variability—"It seems like..." or "Right now, it feels like..."
- impermanence—"Sometimes...," "This time...," and "Currently..."
- hope or possibility—"I can try," "Learning is a process," and "Things can change."

In *being with* practices, we are not seeking to change anything. Being with thoughts involves noticing, naming, and reorienting. You can use this practice yourself, and help guide students to notice, name, and reorient in relation to their thoughts.

1. **Notice** the trauma or protection-based thought—"I can't do this. I can't ever do anything right."
2. **Name** the thought—"That is a trauma-based, personal, negative, and permanent thought."
3. **Reorient:**
   - Reorient to the present moment and the practice—"Right now, I will let that thought be. I am going to focus on my breath, ground my feet, and see what happens."
   - Reorient to a grounding mantra or self-statement—"Right now, I will let that thought be. I know I can try and I am worthy of effort. Being right here and breathing is enough."

Note, Cook-Cottone and colleagues (2017) integrated the body of work on yoga and trauma and consolidated this work into 12 self-statements that aligned with the theory and research. These statements can be very helpful as reorienting thoughts (see Table 14.1).

Table 14.1 Reorienting Self-Statements

Part I: Inner Resources	
Empowerment	I can try
Worth	I am worth the effort
Part II: Physical Basics	
Safety	I deserve to be safe
Breath	My breath is my most powerful tool
Presence	I work toward presence in my body
Feeling	I feel so I can heal
Part III: Self-Regulation	
Grounding	My body is a source for connection, guidance, and coping
Choice	I can find choice in the present moment
Ownership	I can create the conditions for safety and growth
Sustainability	I can create a balance between structure and chance (and effort and rest)
Part IV: Mindful Grit	
Compassion	I honor the individual path of recovery and growth
Self-Determination	I work toward the possibility of effectiveness and growth in my own life

(Informed by Cook-Cottone et al., 2017)

> **Journal Prompt.** Try the noticing, naming, and reorienting thoughts practice. Begin by engaging in a yoga practice in which you pay attention to the thoughts as they move into your awareness. Perhaps in this practice you simply notice them. In another practice, you can notice and name the thoughts. As you build on these skills, you can notice, name, and then practice reorienting. What reorienting mantras or self-statements might you use? How might you use this with your students? How might you cue your students to notice, name, and reorient in relationship to their thoughts?

Shifting to Working with What is Here

Working with is best after time is spent *being with*. You will want to work toward varying lengths of time and types of practice that support being with what is present. Moving to *working with* should be done with awareness, intention, and choice.

Generally, *working with* involves engaging in practices that can help move you up and down the self-regulation scale in service of your wellbeing (see Figure 14.3). This can be formally scheduled—for example, when you offer an energizing vinyasa practice or a restorative yin practice. It can also be done in an attuned manner within an individual session or class. For example, if the class (or person) is showing signs of dysregulation such as irregular breath, sighs, or agitation, you might teach a set of calming practices. If the class (or person) presents as flat, disengaged, listless, you might teach a set of invigorating practices. The goal is attunement and responsiveness to what is present. Chapters 15, 16, and 17 cover a toolbelt of practices to do just that. This imaginary toolbelt has three pockets. The pocket on the left is for calming practices, the one on the right is for energizing practices, and the one in the middle is for balancing practices (practices that are both calming and energizing at the same time).

> **TIR PRINCIPLE: TEACH ATTUNEMENT**
> Teach to noticing sensations, being with what is there, and intentionally choosing being with or working with based on what is noticed.

TEACHING SELF-AWARENESS AND ATTUNEMENT

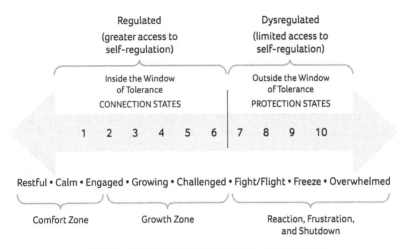

FIGURE 14.3 ENHANCED SELF-REGULATION SCALE

TIR PRACTICE: ATTUNED TEACHING

These categories referred to in Chapters 15, 16, and 17 are not hard and fast rules. They are a good place to start exploring. Each practice is experienced in different ways in different bodies and can serve different roles (calming, activating, or balancing). Generally speaking, you will notice each posture and practice has a target range on the self-regulation scale. This is the range of activation the pose is likely to align with. For example, Warrior 1 is listed in Chapter 15, Practices that Soothe and Calm. For most people, practicing Warrior 1 typically activates around a 3 or a 4 on the self-regulation scale (engaged). If you are feeling challenged (a rating of 5 or 6), Warrior 1 is a calming pose. It offers a stepping stone from activation at 5 or 6, down to 3 or 4. To create a calming sequence, it can be followed by Pyramid Pose (a rating of 3 or 4), Standing Forward Fold (a rating of 2 or 3), and then maybe Child's Pose (a 1 or 2 rating). If you are feeling listless (a rating of 1), a Warrior 1 would be quite energizing (even though we have listed it in Chapter 15). Meeting the mood or activation of the pose and working from there is attuned teaching.

The practices we have included in Chapters 15, 16, and 17 are a combination of ancient and more modern yoga practices developed in the 20th century. There are 56 practices in this book exemplifying the points we make about nervous system regulation. You will find some of the practices are very familiar and some less so. We have chosen these particular poses and breathing practices because they are exemplary of what yoga is about. Along with postures and breathing practices, we offer a few simple meditation practices. Meditation has always been foundational and an integral part of yogic practice, being an invitation to equanimity and calmness (Garner, 2016). Examples of meditation can include body scans, progressive muscle relaxation, seated meditation, visualization, and walking meditation. Spence states, "Over time, your repertoire and comfort level will expand. Each practice can stand alone or be combined with other practices" (2021, p. 48).

Rather than providing a comprehensive way of teaching each practice, the practice chapters (Chapters 15, 16, and 17) provide thoughtful ways to teach particular postures or breathing exercises using TIR methodology. These chapters are designed to serve as a model for an attuned TIR approach. This text is intended to be used to *supplement* 200-, 300-, and 500-hour teacher trainings. There are many, many more postures (asanas), breathing practices (pranayama), sound practice (mantras), and other yoga practices available to you (see Aggarwal, 2020, for an extensive description of yoga practices).

A Note on Contraindications

Know the contraindications for each pose you teach. *Yoga Journal* has an extensive database of yoga poses free to access online. Each pose is listed with a detailed description, and sometimes a video, along with adaptations and contraindications. You can find this at www.yogajournal.com/poses.

You will notice there are no arm- or head-balancing poses in this book. This is deliberate. Although these poses can be beneficial, there are enough contraindications to warrant their exclusion from a text focused on TIR teaching. Additionally, learning for your own practice is not the same as learning to teach those same practices to others. This common misunderstanding has led to many teacher-in-training injuries. Give yourself some grace. There is a lot to learn as you find your way as a new yoga teacher. Focus on what is adaptable and modifiable for your students.

Liability, Insurance, and Permission

Your students will not necessarily know their current health status. This is a good reason to have yoga instructor insurance that covers you wherever you teach, and why insurance liability waivers (where possible) are considered a best practice. The recommendation to check with your doctor before starting (and continuing) a yoga practice (or any physical activity) remains the standard. Check with the place you are teaching. If it is a yoga studio, they probably have a liability waiver and a health condition statement indicating physician approval. If they don't, suggest they get one. Teaching within a medical facility, psychiatric hospital, institution of any kind, or school will require some sort of screening/permission for someone to take your class. This is usually handled within the institution, and you will be informed who is medically cleared to participate in your class. In school settings, children under the age of 18 may need parental approval to participate.

While it may seem like a lot of administrative details have to happen before you begin to teach a class, you only begin once. It is worth the effort to attend to such details and is an important part of professionalizing the process of yoga teaching.

Conclusion

The work of a TIR yoga teacher is to support a yoga student's attunement to and connection with their own bodies through the practices of yoga. After the being with pause, it is time to ground, take a deep breath, and do the next helpful thing. Going forward, you will be exploring yoga practices that can be used to move students up and down the self-regulation scale, out of their comfort zones and into their growth zones, and maintain their ventral vagal connection to self and others.

TEACHER TRAINING DISCUSSION QUESTIONS

1. Why might teaching awareness of and skills for attunement be more effective than simply going slower and calming down?

2. Why learn or teach *being with* skills?

3. What does Viktor Frankl's quote mean to you?

4. How can Warrior I be both a calming and an energizing pose?

5. Why is attention to breathing so critical to your yoga practice and teaching?

CHAPTER 15

Practices that Soothe and Calm

pracchardana-vidhârañâbhyâm vâ prâñasya

Yoga Sutra I:34

Or peace may be reached by the even sending forth and control of the life-breath.

Charles Johnston (1912)

This chapter specifically focuses on practices that soothe and calm the nervous system. These practices can move the nervous system to a state in which the body can be experienced as restful and calm (a blended ventral and dorsal vagal state, with a self-regulation scale rating of 1 or 2). Calming practices can help to dissipate build-up of nervous tension in the body (Spence, 2021). The effect of each practice will vary from student to student. Generally speaking, however, postures with forward flexion of the spine and integration of slower, intentional breathing tend to be calming. There are also other variables to consider as to what makes a practice have a soothing effect including how a student is feeling when they arrive for class, the pace of the practice, and the temperature of the room.

> **TIR PRINCIPLE: PRACTICE IN YOUR PAIN-FREE RANGE OF MOTION**
> Encourage students to move within their pain-free range of motion (staying within the comfort and growth zones).

> **TIR PRINCIPLE:** CONNECT BREATH TO MOVEMENT
> Encourage students to connect breath to movement.

Before we get started, it is important to introduce two principles for practicing within your connection, or ventral vagal state: (1) practice within your pain-free range of motion, and (2) connect breath to movement. Breath holding and dysregulated breath are reliable indicators that you are doing more than you need to in a specific pose. You can only breathe freely and smoothly if you are working within your pain-free range of motion and/or at a pace attuned to your body. Training your students to notice if and when their breath is dysregulated or they are holding their breath will give them real-time data points (signals) about when to pause and do something to create ease in their body. For example, when breath holding and dysregulated breath occurs, it can be helpful to gently ease out of a pose. Do less (or pause) until there is more ease with breath.

> **PRACTICING THE PAUSE**
> Any time, any place, and for any reason, you can always PAUSE. Pause = stop what you are doing, A = assess how you are and what you need, and USE = use your resources.

The added benefit of encouraging students to move in their pain-free range of motion and connect their breath to their movement is that you build how students can care for themselves in every single pose as well as out in the world into your instruction. Small, subtle movements can be powerful. Spence states, "We often overdo it and tell ourselves that a small amount of movement isn't worth the effort. *But it is worth the effort.* Being able to move, even in a small way, is essential to regaining [or building] a fuller range of motion [and experience]" (2021, p. 17).

Note, those who are hypermobile in their joints can find it easier to do yoga poses requiring flexibility. Hypermobility affects about 4–20 percent of the population, tending to decrease with age. Hypermobility correlates with increased risk for injury, joint pain, anxiety, and gut issues. If you (or your students) are hypermobile, it can be more difficult to notice when the body is being pushed too far. You may not get the same range-of-motion cues from your body to pause and hold the stretch where you are. Here lies the risk for injury. For those who are hypermobile, it is important to emphasize drawing into your center and supporting joints when doing calming poses that include folding or bending at joints.

> **Journal Prompt.** As you practice this week, pay attention to your pain-free range of motion, your ability to connect your breath to your movement, and—for those who are hypermobile—the awareness and care of joints. What happens to you as you link your breath to your movement? What happens to your breath when you are experiencing pain or discomfort? Do you notice any patterns across poses or practices?

Props are useful and optional. Encouraging the availability and use of props for your own use as the teacher will serve as a model and demonstration for how props can support your practice. The list below is not exhaustive, but is representative of the most useful and frequently used props in our own teaching settings. That said, there are many occasions when we teach and no props are available (budgetary constraints or no room to store props) or even allowed (in locked facilities like psychiatric hospitals or correctional institutions). When the situation allows, however, we recommend the following props. There are many places where props can be purchased. Depending on the size and quality, the list below can be purchased for under $100. If maintained well, they will last many years. The only thing I (JS) can think of that I have replaced in the last 20 plus years is yoga mats. Generally, props last for decades with normal wear and tear and routine maintenance.

- Yoga mats
- Blankets (thick)
- Foam blocks (about 9 x 6 x 4 inches)
- Strap
- Bolster
- Eye pillow (See Figure 15.1)

Now, it is time to practice. For Chapters 15, 16, and 17, each practice is set up using the English name followed by the Sanskrit name in parentheses. Using both is a way to learn the names of the poses and educate yourself and your students on yoga's language. A brief description of the pose is given along with why you might want to try the pose. This is followed by simple cueing to execute the pose. For some poses, modifications are offered along with the effect it may have on your nervous system. Intentionally, we have only included the essence of the cues without invitational language. It is up to you to integrate the trauma-informed and responsive (TIR) verbal cueing in a way that aligns with the needs of the community within which you teach. As you practice teaching these poses, integrate the invitational language, as well as options related to *being with* and *working with* the pose.

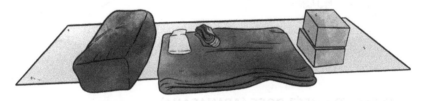

FIGURE 15.1 YOGA PROPS

1. MOUNTAIN POSE (*TADASANA*)

Mountain Pose (Figure 15.2a) offers stability and steadiness. It is the building block for all other standing poses. Standing tall like a mountain also allows for full diaphragmatic breathing that is not possible when your chest is collapsed and your spine slouched.

Mountain Pose begins with the feet hip-width apart with the outside edges of your feet parallel. When you are ready, ground down through the base of the big toe, the little toe, and the outside edge of your feet. Spread and lift the toes slightly. Now let them relax on your mat. Your knees are straight but not locked. Tell yourself "soft knees." Relax your shoulders. Lift your sternum slightly. Let your hands relax by your sides with your fingers pointing down towards the floor. Lift slightly from the crown of your head towards the sky. Relax your face. Release your jaw. Engage your abdominal muscles by gently drawing your navel towards your spine. Mountain Pose is a great check-in pose for your posture and breathing. Try to do it several times a day.

To modify this pose, you can do Chair Mountain Pose (Figure 15.2b). The instruction is the same, except you start from sitting in a solid chair (e.g., a kitchen chair) with your feet hip-width apart, spine straight, sitting with your shoulders over your hips.

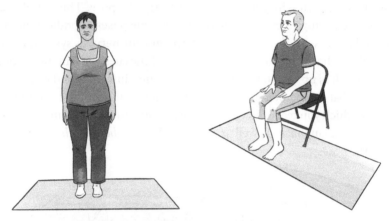

FIGURE 15.2A AND FIGURE 15.2B MOUNTAIN POSE

2. KNEES TO CHEST POSE (*APANASANA*)

Apanasana or Wind-Relieving Pose is a pose for which the English version of the name is something that the pose actually does. It is also okay to use the simple Knees to Chest (Figure 15.3) name. Knees to Chest Pose is helpful to release back tension and can be a very restful pose after a long day.

Begin by lying on your back on your yoga mat. Gently bring your bent knees towards your chest. Place your hands on your knees to guide the movement. Notice how much of your tailbone comes off the mat as you repeat the action. Inhale, allow the knees to move away from the body, and exhale, bring the knees towards the body. Repeat this action three to five times. This pose also can be done one knee at a time.

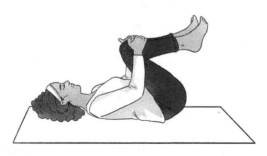

FIGURE 15.3 KNEES TO CHEST POSE

PRACTICES THAT SOOTHE AND CALM

3. LEGS UP THE WALL POSE (*VIPARITA KARANI*)

Legs up the Wall Pose (Figure 15.4a) is a relaxing and soothing pose. The hardest part is getting into it. But when you do, you will want to stay awhile.

Begin on the floor sitting with your hips and shoulders as close to the wall as you can get. Then, as you swing your legs up the wall, allow yourself to lie perpendicular to the wall. You want to get your sitting bones as close to the wall as possible. Notice if your neck is comfortable. If you need some support, use a folded blanket with the minimum amount it takes to feel comfortable. If it feels okay, soften toward the floor. Feel the support of the wall. If you'd like, put your arms in a "T" and rest here for 5–10 minutes. Legs up the Wall Pose will help lengthen your hamstrings. If they are super tight, just taking one leg at a time up the wall is a good idea. To do that, use a door edge so you can let the other leg straighten through the door space (Figure 15.4b).

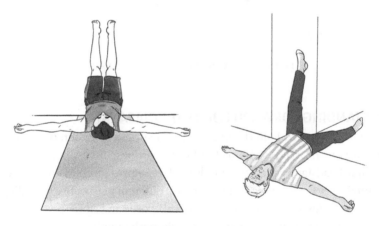

FIGURE 15.4A AND FIGURE 15.4B LEGS UP THE WALL POSE

4. CHILD'S POSE (*BALASANA*)

Child's Pose is a resting pose that invites you to tune inward. Experiment with some props until you find a place of relative ease. This pose is one you will want to try often and return to over and over during your practice time.

Begin on your hands and knees. You can use a folded blanket under your knees. Let your hips move towards your heels, and allow your head to rest on the floor. If your head doesn't easily come to the floor, bring the floor to you. Use a yoga block on the tall end to prop under your forehead (Figure 15.5a). Adjust the block according to your comfort level. If you don't have a block, try stacking your fists one on top of the other, and let your head rest on your stacked fists. If you are using a block for your head, you can let your arms rest beside your body near your feet. Alternatively, you can have your arms outstretched in front of you. Notice your knees and hips. Are you hovering or not able to get comfortable? If you'd prefer, you can try widening the gap between your knees and/or use a bolster placed between your knees. Rest here. Find your breath. Let it be slow and even.

This pose also can be done sitting in a chair (Figure 15.5b). With your hands and arms on a desk, let your head rest on the backs of your hands. Or use a bolster across your lap to support your weight as you drape your body over the bolster. Rest here for several minutes.

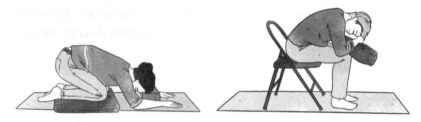

FIGURE 15.5A AND FIGURE 15.5B CHILD'S POSE

5. STANDING FORWARD FOLD (*UTTANASANA*)

Standing Forward Fold (Figure 15.6a) is a simple inversion (your head is below your heart). Inversions tend to be calming. Inversions that do not include headstands and handstands (and therefore less effort and injury) are a simple way to clear your head and gain a different perspective (literally, you are upside down). When starting out, this pose can last for several breaths as a brief taste of an inversion. Eventually, with practice over time, you can work up to 7–8 minutes as a stand-alone refreshing and calming practice.

Begin in Mountain Pose. Then inhale and sweep the arms skyward. As you exhale, hinge forward at the hips. Allow your arms to hang near your feet like a rag doll. The crown of your head is pointing towards the floor. Let your hands rest on something, either a block, the floor, or even your knees or shins. With each inhale and exhale, let your head surrender to the floor. Rest and breathe in the pose. Bending the knees slightly (Figure 15.6b) will help to relieve back strain and hamstring tension. Eventually, you may find less of both in this pose. To come out of the pose, slowly roll up to standing one vertebra at a time until you are vertical. Stand in Mountain Pose and breathe as your body reacclimates to standing upright.

PRACTICES THAT SOOTHE AND CALM

This pose also can be done with your bottom against the wall or sitting on a chair for additional support.

Contraindications: As with any inversion, if you have glaucoma or detached retinas, or if you are pregnant or have unmedicated high blood pressure, this practice is not for you.

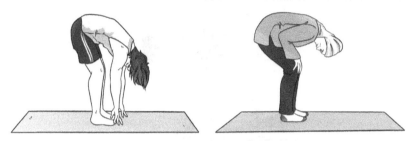

FIGURE 15.6A AND FIGURE 15.6B STANDING FORWARD FOLD

6. RECLINING BOUND ANGLE POSE (*SUPTA BADDHA KONASANA*)

Reclining Bound Angle Pose (Figure 15.7a) is a classic restorative pose that can be restful and energizing at the same time.

Start in Corpse Pose. Bend your knees and place the soles of your feet together and allow the knees to fall away from each other. Place one hand over your heart and the other hand on your belly. Notice if your hips would like more support. If so, slide a block under each knee or a bolster under your knees (Figure 15.7b). If you'd like, rest here for two to five minutes.

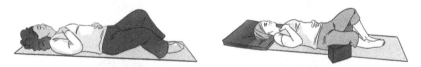

FIGURE 15.7A AND FIGURE 15.7B RECLINING BOUND ANGLE POSE

7. PYRAMID POSE (*PARSVOTTANASANA*)

Pyramid Pose (Figure 15.8) is a standing pose. Begin standing at the top of your mat in Mountain Pose. Step back with one foot about 2–3 feet, allowing your hips to remain square to the front of your mat. If it feels okay, allow the back foot to be at about a 45-degree angle, feet hip-width apart to maintain your balance. From here, with your hands on your hips, hinge forward, keeping your spine long. Pause; breathe. Now gently round your back and gaze towards your knee, placing your hands either on your shins, blocks, or the floor. Find your breath. Press through your feet to come out of the pose, coming up on the inhale. Repeat on the other side. Take a moment to notice the difference. For a simple modification, use a chair instead of blocks. Allow yourself to remain in the pose for several breaths, releasing tension from the face and the backs of the legs.

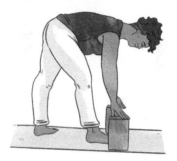

FIGURE 15.8 PYRAMID POSE

8. WARRIOR POSE 1 (*VIRABHADRASANA 1*)

Warrior Pose 1 (Figure 15.9a) is a strong standing pose. It is through the pose's stability that the nervous system is regulated. This pose opens your chest, strengthens your legs, and works your knees and hips.

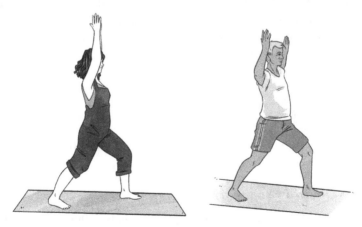

FIGURE 15.9A AND FIGURE 15.9B WARRIOR POSE 1

Begin in Mountain Pose at the top of your mat. Step back with one foot about 2–3 feet, allowing your hips to remain square to the front of your mat.

Allow the back foot to be at about a 45-degree angle, feet hip-width apart to maintain your balance. Your weight is evenly distributed between both feet. As you inhale, draw the arms towards the sky as you bend the front knee. If possible, keep your knee above your ankle. Your back leg is straight and firmly grounded. Soften if you notice any tension or pain. Exhale, staying in the pose with your arms up. Continue to inhale and exhale as you hold the pose. Repeat on the other side.

To be in the pose dynamically, start with both legs straight. Inhale, lift the arms up, exhale, bend the elbows, dropping the arms slightly into a cactus shape (Figure 15.9b), and bend the front knee. Move slowly between having a straight and bent front knee, and lifting and bending the arms three more times. Repeat on the other side.

9. TRIANGLE POSE (*TRIKONASANA*)

Triangle pose (Figure 15.10) is a standing and symmetrical pose. It is a pose of strength and stability.

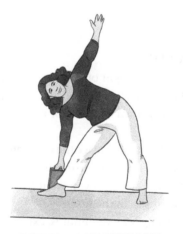

FIGURE 15.10 TRIANGLE POSE

Begin standing in Mountain Pose at the top of your mat. Step back with the left foot about three feet. Allow the left foot to be at about a 45-degree angle. Begin tipping sideways to the right, keeping equal length in the spine. This means *not* collapsing, making one side of the body shorter than the other. Your body and breath will tell you how far to go without straining.

Keep your right leg straight and your knee soft so as not to hyperextend the joint. Let your hand move down your leg towards your knee as your left hand extends towards the sky straight up from your shoulder. Place your right hand on a block or on a chair. The spine is slightly revolved towards the sky as you settle into the pose and find your breath—steady and solid—for about five breath cycles. Adjust the posture as you'd like. Push through your feet to come back to upright and repeat on the other side.

10. BELLY BREATHING

Belly Breathing allows you to completely relax and soften your body. Belly Breathing is simple to do and can be done lying down (Corpse Pose) or sitting (Chair Mountain). While this pose can be done standing in Mountain Pose, it feels more relaxing to have the support of the floor or a chair.

Begin in Corpse Pose. Breathe a regular breath and notice how you are feeling. If you are not breathing through your nose, do so. Place your hands on your belly so you get the added sensory input from your hands. Now start to breathe into your belly. Inhale and feel your belly rise, exhale, feel your belly relax. Repeat this pattern slowly five times. Relax your hands, release the breathing pattern, and breathe a regular breath. Notice how you are feeling.

11. SANDBAG BREATHING

Sandbag Breathing uses the weight of an 8–10-pound sand bag to give you a felt sense of your breath. The weight of the sandbag builds the capacity of your diaphragm—the primary muscle of respiration—as in resistance training.

Begin in Corpse Pose. Carefully place the sandbag either across your hips or across your chest. Note: If you are using an actual sandbag, note which side has a handle grip. If at any time you want to end this practice, gently tug the sandbag and let it slip to the floor.

Practice nasal breathing for two minutes, extending up to five minutes if you feel comfortable and you are breathing easily. Adjust the sandbag to your comfort level (see note above). At the end of the 2–5 minutes, remove the sandbag. Notice how you are breathing. Do you feel the difference? Over time, you will feel more confident in your breathing. This practice can help develop or maintain muscle tone in your diaphragm.

12. SIGHING BREATH

Sighing can serve as a way for the body to dissipate excess nervous energy. Sighing Breath is one of the simplest breathing practices in yoga.

It's one of those practices we tend to do unconsciously or intuitively. Here, we are doing it on purpose with intent. This practice can be done standing, sitting, or lying down. Think of the unconscious sound your breath makes when you get into a hot tub. There's a letting-down response in your nervous system. Sighing intentionally is also a nice way to transition from one section of a class to another, making some noise with your breath, and having some fun at the same time. Eye rolling is optional (Spence, 2021).

Add an arm movement. Inhale, lift the arms, exhale, sigh out through your mouth. Make some noise. Do it two more times.

13. EASY SITTING POSE (*SUKHASANA*)

Easy Sitting Pose (Figure 15.11) is also known as Easy Pose. Some poses do seem easy, but for some, sitting on the floor has never been easy. Learning how to sit comfortably on the floor, at least for a short time, however, is a good skill to have. This pose also can be done in a chair—see Chair Mountain above (Figure 15.2b). This is a resting pose and a good pose for meditation. It is hard to rest and/or meditate and receive the benefits of completing your practice if you do not feel comfortable.

Begin sitting cross-legged on your mat. Sit with your spine straight and your chest lifted. Find a smooth natural breath. Allow your hands to rest comfortably on your knees. If you find yourself slumping or you'd like support, try the following. Use a folded thick blanket; sit on its edge so the blanket is giving support to your tailbone like a small wedge. It will lift your hips. Next, use two blocks, one propped under each knee. After practicing Easy Sitting Pose for some time using props, if it still bothers your knees, hips, or ankles, feel free to try the chair. Remember, the purpose of sitting is steadiness and ease.

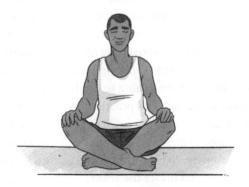

FIGURE 15.11 EASY SITTING POSE

14. NASAL BREATHING

Being able to breathe through one's nose is proven to be superior to mouth breathing. This does not mean mouth breathing is wrong. There are often physical reasons a person is unable to breathe in and out through the nose. This may include having nasal congestion, a deviated septum, or some other sort of nasal blockage. However, mouth breathing could simply be a matter of retraining. This is not hard to do. Nasal breathing warms, humidifies, and filters the air you are breathing. It is a more efficient way to breathe, allowing for a better exchange of carbon dioxide for oxygen. Nose breathers have fewer respiratory infections than mouth breathers (Spence, 2021).

Begin in Mountain Pose, Easy Sitting Pose, or Chair Mountain. Now notice your breath. No need to make any changes. Just notice. If you are not breathing through your nose, see if you can make the switch; if not, just breathe the best you can, slowly and with awareness. Can you purse your lips a little to remind yourself you are breathing through your nose? Can you slow your breath even just a little?

Direct your breath into your diaphragm. To help you locate your diaphragm, place your hands at the bottom of your rib cage and notice the gentle ebb and flow of your breath as your rib cage expands and contracts. Keep going for another 30 seconds or so in a relaxed way. Are you aware of any changes? Notice how you feel in this moment. Is it easy or hard to breathe in and out through your nose? What makes it so? Do you feel your diaphragm moving? Practice nasal breathing anytime you think about it until it becomes your default method of breathing. Remember that your diaphragm is the primary muscle of respiration.

15. STAIR-STEP BREATHING (*VILOMA 1*)

Stair-step breathing is easier than it looks. Often, a busy mind needs something to do. Think of it as giving your dog a bone. Your dog may be quite distracted until you give them a bone; then your dog is quiet and focused. Our minds can be like an enthusiastic dog and need something to latch on to. There is more to this breath than simply breathing in and out through the nose. It gives the mind something to do. Busy minds can find a quiet and focused attention through this practice (Spence, 2021).

Begin sitting in Easy Sitting Pose or Chair Mountain. Take four little sips of air through the nose to make one complete inhalation, as if going up the stairs. Pause for a moment. Exhale as if you are going down an elevator. Do this three times. Pause and notice the effect.

16. RATIO BREATHING

Ratio breathing is a simple and refreshing practice that can be done anywhere at any time. The ratio part refers to the number of seconds you can inhale (the first number), then pausing (or suspending the breath) for a specified number of seconds (the second number), and then exhaling for a specified number of seconds (the third number). You can start with any combination of numbers as long as you end with the highest number. A longer exhale stimulates the parasympathetic branch of the nervous system, calming the nervous system (Spence, 2021).

Begin in Easy Sitting Pose or Chair Mountain. Notice your breathing. We will try 3:2:4 ratio breathing. This means inhale for three seconds, pause for two seconds, and exhale through the nose for four seconds. Practice this pattern for two minutes. Then drop the pattern, breathe in a natural way, and notice the effect.

17. CHANTING OM

The sound "Om," also known as *Aum*, is said to be the original sound at the beginning of creation. "Yoga Sutra 1:28 reminds us that the recitation of that [syllable, OM] [leads to] the contemplation of its meaning" (Johnston, 1912). Om is also considered the most sacred mantra in Hinduism and Tibetan Buddhism, among other faiths (Maharara & Sabar, 2020).

Chanting Om together as a class, either at the beginning or the end, is a unifying practice and brings focus to one's mind. It is also a calming *bija* (meaning seed) sound that is a single syllable mantra from the Sanskrit language first written down in the Vedas, originating between 1500 and 1200 BC (Frawley, 2010). The sound of Om activates the parasympathetic response that relaxes the nervous system. Chanting Om is also a form of co-regulation in that it brings solidarity and oneness as each person in the class breathes and makes sound in unison.

Begin in Easy Sitting Pose. Invite your students to join you in three rounds of the sound of Om if they wish. Take a deep inhale to begin, and exhale while forming the "A" with an open mouth, moving to "u" and "m" as your exhale comes to its natural end and your lips move towards one another until they are closed. Repeat two more times. Listen and feel the oneness of the sound you are making together. Return to a natural breath. Feel the resonance of the sound.

18. CORPSE POSE (SAVASANA)

Resting is part of *every* yoga class. Traditionally and most often, the pose is done lying down. But you also can do the practice sitting if need be. The goal is to do nothing. At all. That is why it is both so easy and so hard. This practice is about your comfort. It is about letting go, which includes letting go of tension from your body and thoughts or patterns of thinking that no longer serve you. It is not even about breathing a certain way. Breathing in any way that is comfortable for you will suffice. When you slow down, you may find some emotions may arise. Sometimes tears appear. Try to welcome what arises. Noticing any arising feelings can be helpful to validate and give expression to something already there.

Practice resting in Corpse daily. Try ten minutes a day (if you can swing it) for a month, and just see what happens. Corpse Pose will help integrate the experience of your yoga practice into your nervous system. This means it can take about 12–14 minutes for your system to down-regulate. During this time of stillness, your body is better able to metabolize the practice you have just done. Using various props is one way to make yourself as comfortable as possible. Use of props is optional but encouraged.

Figure 15.12a (page 234) shows minimal props in Corpse Pose with a folded blanket under the head to support the neck, blocks underneath the backs of the thighs, and an eye pillow over the eyes. Figure 15.12b (page 234) has a more robust use of props including a bolster under the knees; you could also add a blanket over the body, and a weighted sandbag over the abdomen. Each prop you choose to use should be in service of your comfort. If you are not comfortable, you are not going to enjoy Corpse Pose. So, taking the time to gather and set up your props to support your comfort level is well worth the effort. But unless you spell out and give permission for your students to be comfortable, they may not bother, even when many props are at their disposal. It's not hard to imagine that one could easily dismiss Corpse Pose and its accoutrements as fluffy and unnecessary. Nothing could be further from the truth.

A teaching point: if you are using props, before class begins, make the props you think will serve the needs of your students accessible. Have them near your mat in a neat stack so students can see what you will be using at the end of class. Suggest they gather the same props to set aside in preparation for *Savasana*.

Note, lying in *Savasana* with your eyes closed is a relatively vulnerable position. Sometimes individuals who have been through trauma experience distress when asked to lie down and close/cover their eyes. I (CCC) worked

PRACTICES THAT SOOTHE AND CALM

with a yoga student who felt safest doing *Savasana* seated with her back against the wall, oriented toward the entrance, and her eyes open. Some students organize themselves to leave before *Savasana*. Not because they do not value it; rather, it is simply too stressful for them. A TIR yoga teacher is flexible, accepting, and supportive of all the ways yoga students respond to *Savasana*. It can be helpful to remind students to exit quietly to honor the practice of the students staying.

> **Journal Prompt.** Often there is a judgment around people leaving before or during *Savasana*. How is it different when considered from a TIR perspective? What could you do to make sure both the individual who feels they need to leave and those remaining in class have a positive experience?

Lastly, it is very easy to think to yourself, "Just one more pose and then we will quickly do *Savasana* towards the end of a yoga class." Try to resist this thinking. Either your class will run over time or you will be tempted to skip *Savasana*. Neither is good form, etiquette, or practice. So, work backwards as you are planning your class, and allow a minimum of ten minutes of *Savasana* for a 60-minute class or at least 15 minutes for a 75-minute class. There is no hard and fast rule. However, the nervous system takes about 12–15 minutes to physically be able to relax.

Should you talk to your students and give instruction during *Savasana*? It depends on whether your students are new to yoga or not and whether they have practiced *Savasana* before. Perhaps you will know this ahead of time, but perhaps not. A suggestion is to have props out and set up or demonstrate how to use them. You may give a few brief words of instruction. As an example:

> We are practicing "being," not "doing." Breathe any way that feels comfortable to you. If you notice you are thinking, try not to judge the thought, let it go, and come back to your breath. You might simply say to yourself, "thinking." Repeat this as often as you need to. I will keep time and silence for us for the next few minutes. Let yourself rest. Come out of *Savasana* whenever you need to.

Some teachers like to offer soft, slow instrumental music during *Savasana*. This is fine. But do note it is not possible to choose music that will please everyone or not trigger anyone. Perhaps try it both ways with and without music. See what you notice. Is it possible to help your students tune in to the music of their own breathing? Consider what seems to best serve your students.

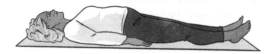

FIGURE 15.12A *SAVASANA* WITH NO PROPS

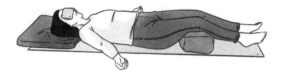

FIGURE 15.12B *SAVASANA* WITH MANY PROPS

> **Journal Prompt.** Do you have a resting practice? What props do you like to use? Or what props would you like to try out? Is resting hard for you? If so, why is that, and how could you make it easier on yourself?

19. MEDITATION

This meditation practice can be done as a stand-alone practice or as part of your class before or after *Savasana*. Sometimes people confuse *Savasana* for Meditation and vice versa. The original intent of asana and pranayama practice is to prepare the body for meditation.

The following is a very simple heart-centered meditation (adapted from Spence, 2021). It can be done sitting on the floor, or on a chair, or lying down. All are fine, although it is usually easier to stay awake if you are sitting. The idea is to be relaxed in your body and alert in your mind. Begin in Easy Sitting Pose. If you would like, place one hand on your heart and one hand on your belly. Notice your breath. Notice the sensation and weight of your hands making contact with your body. Perhaps you can feel your heart beating. Deepen your breath. Perhaps you can feel the rise and fall of your belly. Feel free to have your eyes open or closed, whichever feels better to you. If your eyes are open, see if you can soften your gaze.

Notice your hands again. This gesture of placing the hand on the heart is often a gesture of comfort or wholeheartedness, and that's what you are communicating nonverbally to yourself right now. These gestures are a way for you to comfort and care for yourself in this moment. Recognize that your heart is beating under your hand. Perhaps you can feel the beating of your heart.

Whether or not you can feel your heart beating, sense the work of your heart. It works on your behalf without you even thinking about it. A beating heart is one of the many automatic functions of your amazing body. Just know that, in this moment, your heart is doing its job.

As you hold your hand over your heart, see your heart in your mind's eye, pumping, working hard, taking care of business for you, moment by moment. Be aware of the heart's inner working, steadily beating under your hand. Perhaps this action evokes gratitude. Recognize it if it is there.

Shift your awareness to your belly. Sometimes our breathing is deep enough to move the belly. Notice the rise and fall of your belly as you breathe in and out through your nose.

Our ability to care for ourselves is vital to our wellbeing. That's what you are doing for yourself right now, in this moment—being aware of and caring for yourself. Notice how it feels to do this for yourself. No one can do this work for you. Only you can do it for yourself.

Perhaps remain still and quiet for a minute or so. Let your hands relax by your sides. Notice the absence of your hands from your body, the change of pressure. Remember your hands' capacity for kindness. Are there other people to whom these hands can be kind? If your eyes are closed, open them. Orient yourself to the room. Notice your breathing.

TEACHER TRAINING DISCUSSION QUESTIONS

1. Name three poses in English and in Sanskrit that can calm the nervous system and describe how you might integrate them into a yoga class or session.

2. Name elements of each of the three poses that contribute to the calming effect.

3. Should *Savasana* be part of every yoga class? Why or why not?

4. Is there a practice in this chapter that you gravitate to? Why is that?
5. What props do you find most helpful for calming and soothing poses? Describe why and how you like to use them.
6. What props might you offer someone who is visibly uncomfortable in Easy Sitting Pose?

CHAPTER 16

Practices that Activate and Stimulate

sthira-sukham âsanam

Yoga Sutra II:46

Right poise [asana] must be firm [alert] and without strain [relaxed].

Charles Johnston (1912)

There is much advice written about our need to de-stress and calm down to have a better life. A regular yoga practice can certainly contribute to how we do that. It is also important to understand that an activated nervous system is not the enemy and is often very helpful. According to the polyvagal theory, a highly activated nervous system responds to protect you. In daily life, activation at this level can be stressful and problematic. In many of our daily life tasks, however, we need to be energized in a regulated way. In this blended state, the ventral vagal complex and sympathetic nervous system are activated. We refer to this as the growth zone; yoga students are engaged, growing, and challenged without being overly activated (e.g., outside of the window of tolerance and in flight or flight). We use this type of activation to get ourselves up and out of bed in the morning, gear up to teach a yoga class, and learn a new practice or posture. Energizing practices work well to help you wake up in the morning or to reinvigorate you during your mid-afternoon slump when your energy naturally drops.

Note that cardiovascular effort does not dictate the energizing quality of a pose or breathing practice. Each will have a different effect and require different effort. Some practices look so simple. Considering the small amount of movement in some practices, you may wonder how it could be stimulating to your nervous system. Think of Bellows Breath as an example—done without the arm movement, the only visible movement is the rib cage expanding and contracting. Yet, after just ten inhales and exhales, you will notice an increase in your pulse rate as if you were taking a brisk walk. Doing Bellows Breath is not a replacement for taking a brisk walk—something you may want to do daily—but it reveals important information about how powerful your breathing is when you harness it. The application of this knowledge will revolutionize your life.

You may find many of the poses below can be done dynamically and/or statically and may or may not be physically challenging for you. Dynamic in this case means there may be movement within the pose and that movement is coordinated with the breath, whereas a static pose may be held in stillness while also paying attention to your breath.

1. HORSE WHINNY

This practice is aptly named; it sounds just like a horse whinnying. It is fun, expressive, and easy. The longer inhale helps energize clients by stimulating the sympathetic branch of the autonomic nervous system, followed by a comparatively shorter exhale (or whinny). This is a good practice to do anytime you notice excessive tension in your students' faces (or your own).

Begin in Mountain Pose. Become aware of tension in your face. In your jaw? Your eyes? Your cheeks?

Inhale slowly through the nose, and then on the exhale, purse your lips together and make a horse or motor sound, quickly pushing the air through your pursed lips. Now add raising your arms over your head on the inhale, and dropping them down to your side on your exhale. Notice tension releasing from your face.

2. BELLOWS BREATH (*BHASTRIKA PRANAYAMA*)

Bellows Breath is named after the old-fashioned bellows used to fan the flame in the fireplace. It is a reliable way to excite the nervous system. You may notice an immediate elevation of your heart rate. Therefore, unless you are an advanced pranayama practitioner (as in having many years of practice under your belt), less than one minute of this practice is recommended. The preferred length is about ten inhales and exhales. This is a seated practice only.

Caution: If you have unmedicated high blood pressure, shoulder issues, or you are feeling quite anxious, this practice is not for you.

Begin in Easy Sitting Pose or Chair Mountain. Notice your breathing. There are two parts to this practice that can be done together or separately. To practice the breathing part, try a quick passive inhale through the nose followed by a forceful exhale through the nose. Repeat. For the arm movement, begin with the hands at chest height and make a fist, letting your fingers wrap around your thumbs. Then on your next inhale, move your hands skywards, leading with your fingers. On the exhale, draw the arms down to the starting position (fingers curled around your thumbs) as in Figure 16.1. This arm movement simulates a gentle pumping action allowing lymph to flow better in your body.

Coordinate your breathing with the arm movement for ten repetitions. Follow with two slow arm movements. Let your hands rest in your lap. Sense into your right hand, sense into your left hand. Sense into your right foot, sense into your left foot. Notice the effect of the practice.

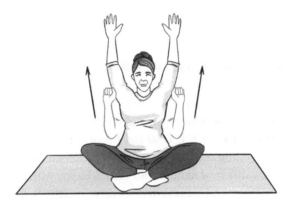

FIGURE 16.1 BELLOWS BREATH

3. WARRIOR POSE 2 (*VIRABHADRASANA 2*)

Warrior poses are strong, grounding poses. They help you to take up space and stand firm, not unlike power posing.

Begin in Mountain Pose, standing at the top of your mat. Step back about 3-4 feet with as much width between the feet as you need to feel balanced and grounded. The back foot is at a 45-degree angle. Your weight is evenly distributed between each foot. Inhale and bend the front knee, allowing the knee to remain stacked over the heel. Exhale as you lift the arms parallel to the floor. If your right knee is forward, stretch your right arm in front of your chest and the left arm directly behind you, both at shoulder height. Your chest is lifted, and your gaze (*drishti*) is over your second or third finger as in Figure 16.2. Again, feel your feet on the floor. Hold the pose and breathe for three breath cycles. To come out of the pose, step your back foot into Mountain Pose or simply unbend your knee and relax your arms. Notice the effort.

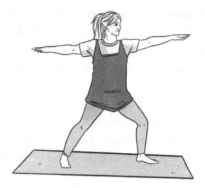

FIGURE 16.2 WARRIOR POSE 2

4. REVERSE WARRIOR POSE (*VIPARITA VIRABHADRASANA*)

Reverse Warrior Pose adds a vulnerability or softness to the Warrior Pose. The vulnerability added by lifting and reaching through one arm can be energizing as you feel that side of the body open and your drishti moves upward.

Begin in Warrior Pose 2. If your right foot is forward, lift your right arm towards the ceiling and ease into a slight backbend. Your hand is like a mirror—gaze towards your hand if your neck is happy with this movement as in Figure 16.3. Pause and breathe here for three breaths. Return to Warrior Pose 2. Straighten your leg. Rest and breathe. Repeat on the other side.

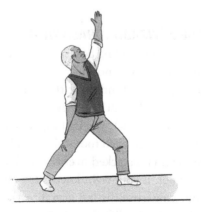

FIGURE 16.3 REVERSE WARRIOR POSE

PRACTICES THAT ACTIVATE AND STIMULATE

5. MODIFIED SIDE ANGLE POSE (*PARSVAKONASANA*)

Modified Side Angle Pose is another strong, grounding pose. It is also activating. Your feet press into the floor and your core is activated, supporting the extension of the spine and the reaching of your hand.

Begin in Warrior Pose 2 with the right leg forward. Inhale to prepare, then exhale and tilt your body to the right until your right elbow rests comfortably on your thigh. If your elbow does not go easily on your thigh as in Figure 16.4a, put your hand on your thigh as in Figure 16.4b. Pause. Inhale as you rotate your spine slightly toward the ceiling. Now, lift your left arm above the shoulder also towards the ceiling. Pause and exhale. Remain here for three more breaths. Alternatively, you can inhale, taking your right arm toward the front of your mat, creating a long, curved line from your fingertips to your heel. Exhale. Pause and remain here or allow your arm to rest along the side of your body for three breath cycles. To come out of the pose, inhale to prepare, exhale and bring your body upright, relax your arms, straighten your right leg, and breathe. Repeat on the other side.

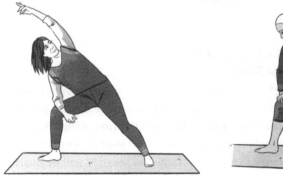
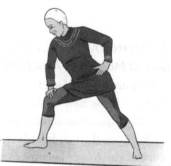

FIGURE 16.4A AND FIGURE 16.4B MODIFIED SIDE ANGLE POSE

6. CHAIR POSE (*UTKATASANA*)

Chair Pose is a standing pose. It activates large muscle groups in the legs, hips, and glutes. Your heart is tasked with fueling these muscles with oxygen, and this is experienced by most as a demanding pose. It can increase your strength and endurance.

Begin in Mountain Pose. Slowly bend your knees as if you are going to sit on a chair as in Figure 16.5. Your quads will immediately activate. This physically demanding pose will require much practice to allow your breath to be smooth and even. Start off with small—rather than deep—bending of the knees. Increase your effort/stamina over time. The pose can be held statically for five to ten rounds of breath. Or the pose can be practiced dynamically with raising the arms above the head on the inhale and sinking into the pose on the exhale, knees bent, arms outstretched and forward.

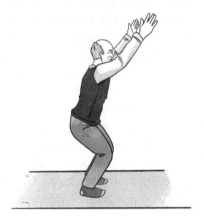

FIGURE 16.5 CHAIR

7. DOWNWARD-FACING DOG POSE (*ADHO MUKHA SVANASANA*)

Downward-Facing Dog Pose asks a lot of your body. It is full of effort, especially for those new to the pose. It is also an inversion and, with practice, you may experience sensations of strength and relaxation at the same time.

Begin on the hands and knees on all fours. Curl your toes under. Placement of the hands becomes very important now, as they will be bearing your weight. Hands are flat, spread out, and placed shoulder-width apart (or even a little wider than the shoulders). Inhale, lift your hips toward the ceiling into an upside-down "V" as in Figure 16.6a. This pose will strengthen your inhale and your exhale.

Allow your head to be relaxed, with no tension in the neck. Outwardly rotate your shoulders (without moving your hand position). Lengthen your spine on the inhale, pushing down through your arms and into your hands as you lift your hips. As you exhale, focus on lengthening the backs of the legs. Your heels may not be on the floor, but they are heading in that direction. Bend your knees if your back is rounding as in Figure 16.6b. Stay here for several rounds of inhales and exhales. Enjoy that your head is being supported by your hands and feet. Come out of the pose and rest in Child's Pose. This pose can also be done with your hands against the wall or with

PRACTICES THAT ACTIVATE AND STIMULATE

your hands on a chair (as in Figure 16.6c) if you have shoulder concerns or weight-bearing with your hands feels too taxing on your shoulders.

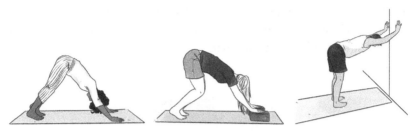

FIGURE 16.6A, FIGURE 16.6B, AND FIGURE 16.6C DOWNWARD FACING DOG

8. UPWARD-FACING DOG POSE (*URDHVA MUKHA SVANASANA*)

Upward-Facing Dog Pose is an energizing pose that stretches the chest and spine, while strengthening the wrists, arms, and shoulders.

Begin in Cobra Pose. Then draw the elbows close to your body with hands flat on the floor in line with your chest. Inhale, lift your chest upwards until your arms are straight, and allow your knees to rise off the floor. Keep length in your spine and neck without crunching the spine as in Figure 16.7a. Exhale, lower your chest and knees back to the floor. Repeat three times, then rest in Child's Pose. Alternatively, this pose can be done while keeping your knees on the floor as in Figure 16.7b.

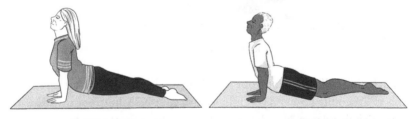

FIGURE 16.7A AND FIGURE 16.7B UPWARD-FACING DOG POSE

9. REVERSE TABLE TOP POSE (*ARDHA PURVOTTANASANA*)

Reverse Table Top Pose can open up the entire front side of the body in an energizing way. This pose will provide a deep stretch to the shoulders, chest, abdomen, and spine. It will build strength throughout the core muscles and those surrounding the spine. It will strengthen the wrists, arms, buttocks, legs, and back.

Begin sitting belly up on your mat. Place your hands shoulder-width apart under your shoulders. Fingers are pointing towards your body. Feet are hip-width apart; knees are bent. Inhale, lift your hips towards the ceiling until you resemble a table top (Figure 16.8). Your head will naturally tilt back. Your chest will be open. Exhale, return to the mat. Repeat five times and rest sitting or lying on your mat.

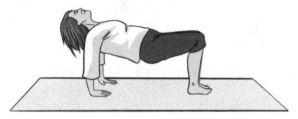

FIGURE 16.8 REVERSE TABLE TOP POSE

10. BABY COBRA POSE (*ARDHA BHUJANGASANA*)

Baby Cobra Pose (Figure 16.9) is a backbend that both energizes the body and strengthens the back. This is an important pose for long-term care of your back.

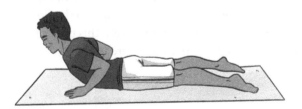

FIGURE 16.9 BABY COBRA POSE

Begin facing belly down on your mat. Let your head rest on your forearms. This is Crocodile Pose. As you inhale, pull your belly button towards your spine. Exhale release. Now let your elbows help support your body weight, with palms down. With the chin tucked slightly, inhale and lift your chest; your legs and feet extend away from your body as shown in Figure 16.9. Exhale. Stay here in the pose for three more breaths, then rest with your head on your forearms.

To do the pose dynamically, let your hands rest flat on your mat and lined up under each shoulder. Inhale, and slowly push into your hands, allowing your breath and your abs to float your body upwards. Elbows remain bent. For the next three breaths, inhale upwards and exhale back to

PRACTICES THAT ACTIVATE AND STIMULATE

the mat. Allow your arms to be passive and focus your effort in your breath and your back. Come up only as high as is comfortable. This pose is more about stretching the front of the body than bending the back. Remember, less is more. Don't force your back to bend. Be gentle. Even small, mindful backbends are effective. End as you began by resting in Crocodile Pose.

11. BLOCK BREATHING

Sometimes we hold a lot of tension in our diaphragms—the primary muscle of respiration. This pose provides compression of the diaphragm and will help you identify and release that tension. Start slowly and be kind to yourself. Let your arms and shoulders support some of your body weight. You may need to build up to two minutes. The end result will be a fuller exhalation.

Start in Cobra Pose. Place a yoga block centered under the belly button (or improvise with a book). You can control the amount of body weight you are placing on the block by at first using bent elbows to disperse your weight (Figure 16.10). Palms are facing down.

Do this for two minutes or to your tolerance level. There may be some discomfort at first and you may feel your aorta pulsating strongly. As you inhale fully, pause and focus on exhaling fully. Then pause and repeat. At the end of two minutes, remove the block and notice your breathing. Rest in Hero Pose or Child's Pose.

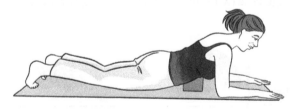

FIGURE 16.10 BLOCK BREATHING

12. LOCUST POSE (*SALABHASANA*)

This fun pose is sometimes called Superwoman/Superman Pose. It is an excellent pose for strengthening the spine. You may want to practice this pose with a folded blanket under your pelvis.

Begin face down, head on the mat, and your arms stretched out over your head but touching the floor. One variation is to lift the left arm and your right foot at the same time as in Figure 16.11a. To do this, inhale and bring your belly button towards your spine. Exhale. Inhale, lift your left arm and right foot off the mat. Your chest is lifting off the mat too. Exhale back down. Repeat for three more breaths. Then rest. For the second variation, lift both hands and legs off the mat at the same time as in Figure 16.11b. Inhale, lift, exhale down.

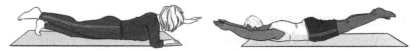

FIGURE 16.11A AND FIGURE 16.11B LOCUST POSE

13. BRIDGE POSE (*SETU BANDHASANA*)

Bridge Pose is a backbending pose that has many variations. It stretches and opens the front of the body and strengthens the back of the body. It can be done actively or passively and is a good counter to slouching or sitting for long periods of time.

Begin in Corpse Pose. Bend your knees, lift your hips, and place a block under your hips as in Figure 16.12a. Take a few breaths here and notice the angle of your pelvis. Another version of Bridge Pose is to take the block away and move dynamically with the breath from Bridge Pose while returning the hips and back to the mat as in Figure 16.12b. As you exhale back down to your mat, allow your arms to move over your head. A third variation is to hold Bridge Pose (without the block) and simply breathe.

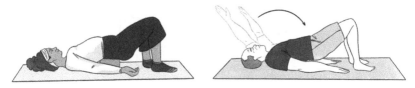

FIGURE 16.12A AND FIGURE 16.12B BRIDGE POSE

14. MODIFIED CAMEL POSE (*USTRASANA*)

Camel Pose is a backbending pose. Camel Pose has variations according to your energy level and backbending ability today. Camel Pose is stimulating and opens the front line of the body.

Begin kneeling. Feel free to place a folded blanket under your knees. Place your hands on your lower spine or the lower glutes for support. Inhale to elongate the spine and continue into extension (a backbend) until you

PRACTICES THAT ACTIVATE AND STIMULATE

get to the end of your inhale, or you feel the natural end-range of your back bend. Your head and neck are going along for the ride. Pause for a few beats. As you exhale, return to a neutral spine and let your chin move towards your chest. This is the dynamic version of Camel Pose. To do the pose statically, inhale and gently extend the spine as in Figure 16.13. Pause. Exhale and remain in extension for three breaths. Exhale to return to a neutral spine. Take a few breaths in Child's Pose.

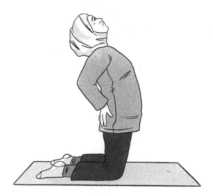

FIGURE 16.13 MODIFIED CAMEL POSE

15. PLANK POSE (*KUMBHAKASANA*)

Plank Pose is an energizing pose that strengthens the entire body. It builds isometric strength simply by using your body weight.

Begin on all fours on your mat. Place your hands underneath your shoulders. Your hands are flat and spread out. Extend each leg and balance on curled toes as in Figure 16.14a. Find your breath. If you are holding your breath, let your knees rest on the floor as in Figure 16.14b. Take three rounds of breathing. Return to all fours and rest in Child's Pose.

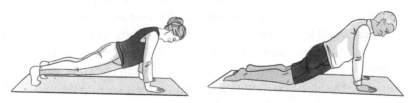

FIGURE 16.14A AND FIGURE 16.14B PLANK POSE

16. SIDE PLANK POSE (*VASISTHASANA*)

Side Plank Pose is a challenging arm balance that strengthens the entire body. Much like Plank Pose, it builds isometric strength by simply using your body weight.

Begin in Plank Pose (see above), pause, and breathe. Inhale, as you stack one foot on top of the other and rotate your body upwards, taking your weight onto one hand as in Figure 16.15a. Exhale. Find your balance. Find your breath. Breathe here for three breaths. If you want, place your upper foot on the mat in front to take some tension off your shoulder. Come out of the pose and rest on your belly. Repeat on the other side. An alternative way to do Side Plank Pose is resting on your forearm with a bent elbow (instead of your hand). Your elbow will be lined up underneath your shoulder. Your other hand can provide balance in front of your body placed on the mat as in Figure 16.15b.

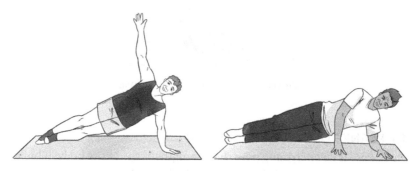

FIGURE 16.15A AND FIGURE 16.15B SIDE PLANK POSE

17. CRESCENT LUNGE POSE (*ANJANEYASANA*)

This simple lunge can feel good on your hips. It is an asymmetrical pose that requires a release of hip tension when using the front foot and a stretching of the psoas (a major hip flexor) on the other side. The pose can be done with the knee on or off the mat and with different arm positions.

Begin on all fours. Bring the left foot forward and place between your hands, allowing your foot to rest comfortably in line with your knee as in Figure 16.16a. Use blocks either side of your foot to rest your hands on if you want. Decide if you want to stay with your left knee on the mat or lift it up. Or you can move between knee on the mat and knee off the mat, coordinating with your breath. As a variation, you can either keep your hands on the blocks or raise them over your head with your palms facing inward as in Figure 16.16b. Stay here for several breaths.

PRACTICES THAT ACTIVATE AND STIMULATE

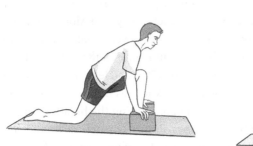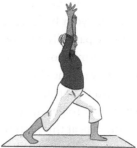

FIGURE 16.16A AND FIGURE 16.16B CRESCENT LUNGE POSE

18. BOAT POSE (*NAVASANA*)

Boat Pose strengthens the core. It works the deep hip flexors. It is also a balancing pose.

Begin sitting in Staff Pose (sitting up straight with your legs out in front of you). Inhale and slowly draw your legs upwards with your knees bent until you are balancing on your sitting bones with your hands clasping the back of your thighs as in Figure 16.17a. Exhale. On your next inhale, straighten your legs out in front of you. Exhale. If you are able to maintain your balance here, inhale and extend your arms either side of each leg. Balance here for three more breaths. To come out of the pose, put your feet on the mat and slowly recline to the floor. Alternatively, keep your knees bent and your hands under your thighs as in Figure 16.17b. Balance here for several breaths.

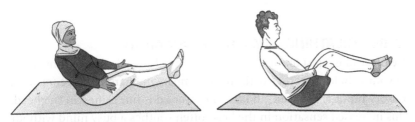

FIGURE 16.17A AND FIGURE 16.17B BOAT POSE

19. BREATH OF JOY

Breath of Joy is a great way to wake yourself up in the morning and elevate your mood. Some use it as a caffeine alternative for that mid-afternoon energy slump. Use this pose when an energy boost or release is needed.

This pose is a standing practice, but you can do it sitting if that would be more comfortable. Either way, you will need plenty of room to move your arms out from your body like a music conductor. Begin in Mountain Pose. As you inhale partially, lift your arms up to chest level. Inhale a little more and let your arms move out to each side as in Figure 16.18a. Inhale, lifting your arms toward the sky. Then exhale with a "ha" and let your arms swing down toward the ground as you bend your knees as in Figure 16.18b. Do it slowly at first to get the mechanics of coordinating the breath with the movement. Repeat this pattern three times. Return to a natural in-and-out breath through the nose. What do you notice? Has your energy shifted? Do you need to catch your breath?

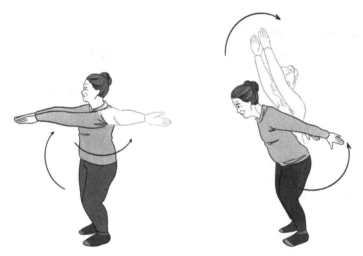

FIGURE 16.18A AND FIGURE 16.18B BREATH OF JOY

20. BEE BREATHING (*BHRAMARI PRANAYAMA*)

Bee Breathing is just like it sounds and is named after the "zzz" sound made on your exhale. Together with the accompanying hand gesture (*mudra*), sensory input is reduced, and the "zzz" sound is intensified in the head. This increased sensation in the head often soothes a busy mind without overstimulating it. This practice can be both calming and energizing at the same time. Note what it is for you.

First, the breathing part of the practice. Begin in Easy Sitting Pose or Chair Mountain. Inhale slowly. On your exhale, begin making the "zzz" sound. It's okay if your lips come apart slightly. The hand gesture is as if you are putting a mask on your face using your hands as the mask. Thumbs are pushing the cartilage gently into the ear; index fingers rest on your brow;

middle fingers rest on your closed eyelids; ring fingers rest at the edge of the nostrils; little fingers rest at the edge of your mouth as in Figure 16.19a. To begin, drop your chin, inhale, and exhale "zzz." After the third time, rest your hands in your lap. If you are practicing in a group, wait for others to finish. Sense your right hand, sense your left hand, sense your right foot, sense your left foot. Open your eyes if they are still closed. Feel free not to use the above hand mudra and just do the breathing part. Or use Helmet Mudra as in Figure 16.19b. This is done by placing your hands on your head and letting your fingers overlap slightly as if your hands are forming a helmet on your head.

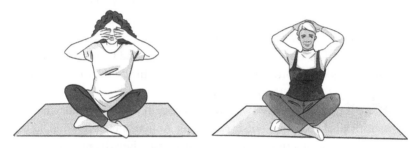

FIGURE 16.19A AND FIGURE 16.19B BEE BREATHING

21. LION'S BREATH (*SIMHASANA*)

Lion's Breath (Figure 16.20) is a good practice to help someone find their voice. It can also release tension in the face and throat. This pose can be done sitting on the floor or a chair (or even in the car if you want to scare nearby motorists!). Lion's Breath is an easy way to energize yourself and release upper-body tension.

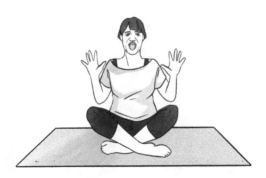

FIGURE 16.20 LION'S BREATH

Begin in Easy Sitting Pose or Chair Mountain with your hands resting on your thighs. Notice your breathing. Your spine is straight. When you are ready, open your eyes wide, look up, and, on the next inhale, lift your hands in front of your chest, spreading the fingers wide like stars. Exhale, making a fairly forceful "ha" sound while sticking your tongue out as in Figure 16.20. Relax your hands and rest them on your legs. Repeat two more times. Relax your body and your face. Notice how you feel.

22. SHAKING

This practice is best done standing. If Shaking is sustained for two or more minutes, you will feel your nervous system revving up. The practice is done gently and mindfully. You are not trying to rattle your brain out of your head. It takes a surprising amount of energy and focus to sustain this practice and is well worth the effort. Like most things, the more you do it, the easier it is to find a rhythm to the practice.

There is no hard and fast way to shake. Begin with the hands, then the arms, until all of your upper body is shaking. At first, it is easier to shake one part of your body at a time. Try one leg at a time, then the hips, shoulders. Your movement here is understated—small, smooth, and full of ease. Be gentle with yourself.

23. STANDING SQUAT POSE (*UTKATA KONASANA*)

Standing Squat Pose (Figure 16.21), also known as Goddess Pose, is a wide-leg standing pose that strengthens the lower body and opens the hips. This pose warms and energizes the body.

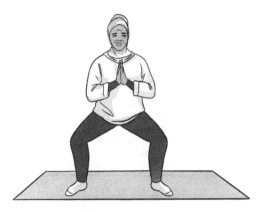

FIGURE 16.21 STANDING SQUAT POSE

Begin in Mountain Pose. Step your feet three to four feet apart. Angle your toes towards the corners of your mat. Inhale to prepare, then as you exhale, start to sink your tail bone towards the floor. Let your knees bend over your toes. Find a comfortable stopping point. Bring your hands together at your heart center as in Figure 16.21. Breathe here for five breaths. Keep your face, jaw, and shoulders soft. Notice the effort. Push through your feet to come out of the pose.

24. MEDITATION

This meditation practice can be done as a stand-alone practice or as part of your class, before or after *Savasana*. The following guided meditation (adapted from Spence, 2021) can be done sitting on the floor, sitting on a chair, or lying down. All are fine, although it is usually easier to stay awake if you are sitting. The idea is to be relaxed in your body and alert in your mind.

Find a comfortable position with your back straight. Feel free to have your eyes open or closed. If they are closed, gaze at the back of your eyelids if you want. It is often easier to do this practice with your eyes closed. If closing your eyes is not comfortable for you today, simply soften your gaze. This practice is about noticing your inner speed and slowing it down. Sometimes, even when we can move slowly on the outside, we are speeding along on the inside.

Begin noticing your breath. What is the length of your breath?

Imagine you are a car traveling down a highway. Notice what sort of car you are. If you own a car, maybe it is a car like that or maybe it is your dream car. How fast do you think you are going as you travel down the highway? Look at your car's dashboard—did you guess correctly? What is the speedometer telling you? Note the speed. How does it feel? Take some time in silence.

What would it feel like to go ten miles per hour slower? How does that feel? Take some time in silence.

What about 20 miles per hour slower? How does that feel? Take some time in silence.

What about slowing down to half speed? How does that feel? Take some time in silence.

Can you slow down even more? What are you noticing at this new, slow pace? Take some time in silence.

Now increase your speed to a pace that feels comfortable for you. Consider maintaining this speed for the rest of your trip. Take some time in silence.

Start slowing down again. You are nearly at your destination. You are just a few blocks from home. You see your parking space. Now you are at your front door.

Notice how it feels to have taken a leisurely drive home. Was it your usual pace? Was it annoying or freeing to slow down? How did your breath respond to this imaginative exercise?

How do you feel now?

Journal Prompt. Is there a yoga posture or breathing practice that you find stimulating to your sympathetic nervous system? How does this practice feel when you practice it? Are you naturally drawn to a particular practice in the morning? Do you have a time in your day when your energy slumps a little? What is your go-to practice when your energy slumps? What else could you try?

TEACHER TRAINING DISCUSSION QUESTIONS

1. Name three poses in English and in Sanskrit that can stimulate the nervous system.

2. Name elements of each of the three poses that contribute to the stimulating effect.

3. Should breathing practices be part of every yoga class? Why or why not?

4. Why is it important to know how to stimulate the nervous system? When is such knowledge useful?

CHAPTER 17

Practices that Balance and Integrate

tato dvandvânabhighâtaï

Yoga Sutra II:48

The fruit of right poise [asana] is the strength to resist the shocks of infatuation or sorrow.

Charles Johnston (1912)

Balance can mean several things. A pose such as Tree Pose is about putting all your weight on one foot, while lifting the other, which, of course, is a pose highlighting the physical balancing of one's body weight. There are also practices that balance energy, increase energy when it is flagging, or decrease energy when we need to unwind and rest. In this chapter, the word *balance* is also used interchangeably with the word *integrate*. The body needs frequent pauses for the new information from a practice to connect with your nervous system. As you take a beat and rest or breathe (or both), your body gets a chance to notice the effect of a practice and for the practice to become part of your general body awareness. Balance and integration are markers of being within your window of tolerance and activation of the ventral vagal complex. To achieve balance and integration, the body and mind connect. Neurologically, the hemispheres of the brain, the areas responsible for coordination of movement, and the emotional and cognitive areas are activated in self-regulating patterns.

Balancing poses can help you notice when your energy is fluctuating—physically, emotionally, or both. Irregular states of energy may be a signal you need to take a break and rest, or that you need a balancing practice to even out your energy or find your equilibrium again. As an example, when you have too much energy, you may feel anxious, and there are calming practices that you can use. Or when you feel flat and lethargic, there are practices that can help you to feel more energized. Even so, each practice can feel different at different times and with different people. There is not a one-size-fits-all effect for each practice.

As a reminder, some of the practices below could just as logically be placed in the chapters on calming practices or energizing practices. This is why practice over time will help you to understand how the practices affect you as the teacher. An example of such a practice is Alternate Nostril Breathing. In the case of Alternate Nostril Breathing, this practice can be both calming and balancing at the same time. The fun is in exploring and developing your awareness as you go along. Be curious. Try pausing at the end of any practice to notice the effect rather than rushing on to the next one. Over time, you will begin to notice the effect of particular practices on your students (and on you) and help them to connect to their own experience.

If practicing a balancing pose (such as Tree Pose, or Dancer Pose) is difficult—if you are unable to balance and stay in the pose for more than a breath or two—the pose may also give you information on your mental state in the moment. Perhaps you are upset or agitated, even though you were previously unaware that you were upset or agitated. This is important information to note. Shirley Telles, director of the Patanjali Research Foundation, says, "Yoga teaches a person to live in harmony, where there is a balance within themselves, and in their emotions and their intellect" (Telles, n.d.). In this way, perhaps consider whether you want to go into a meeting of significance or have a conversation involving high stakes feeling agitated and unsettled. Probably not. A pose like Tree Pose can become an easy way to check in and tune in to yourself physically and mentally. This check-in information can then give you information and options. Do I need to calm or soothe myself right now? Could Nasal Breathing or Ratio Breathing for a few minutes allow your prefrontal cortex—the brain's executive function center (where decision making comes from)—to come back online? The more you practice checking in and tuning in, the easier it gets to notice how you are doing and whether you want to do anything about it. Note, sometimes *being with* how you are doing in the moment is enough.

Many years ago when I (JS) was learning to teach yoga to children, my teacher, Leah Kalish, in her effort to help us be more child-like, used the metaphor of a jungle gym. I remember both loving and fearing the jungle gym as a child. I loved it because I could climb high and still get back down easily, and I could hang upside down. These were also my fears—fear of heights and of falling on my head. Leah reminded us that yoga was like a playground for adults and children. Since then, I have been able to better appreciate Downward-Facing Dog Pose and Standing Forward Fold as my playground for hanging upside down without the fear of falling, and it feels amazing. It is important to integrate joy and play in trauma-informed and responsive (TIR) work. Trauma and stress can block our access to joy. When working with, or perhaps playing with, balance and integrating poses, trying and falling out of the pose can feel a lot like the play of children. In the ventral vagal, connection states, we try hard things, smile or laugh with our failed attempts, and simultaneously open a window of access to joy.

> **Journal Prompt.** After your next practice, consider these questions. What did you notice about your balance? Did you feel steady, shaky? How do you know you are balanced? During the practice, did you feel integration, a coming together of awareness, breath, movement, and your energy? How do you know you are integrated? In the trying, did you notice any joy? In what ways can your experiences with these poses and your own access to joy inform your TIR teaching?

1. TREE POSE (*VRKSASANA*)

Tree Pose is a favorite of ours and a staple of nearly every children's class I (JS) have ever taught. It always feels good to do Tree Pose with an actual tree in your sight lines. Trees have their own healing properties and interconnectedness to their surroundings. Emulating a tree is fun. It also gives you information about the state you are in. Have you ever noticed how hard it is to balance on one foot when you are feeling upset or angry?

Begin by standing in Mountain Pose. Lift one foot to rest against the inside of the other leg. Your foot can rest above the knee on the inside surface of the thigh (as in Figure 17.1a), just not on the knee joint itself—placement here creates too much pressure on the knee joint. You can choose to hold on to a chair or bring your hands together at your heart center. Or instead of lifting your foot, simply lift your heel off the floor, letting your toe remain on the floor as in Figure 17.1b, more like a Sapling Pose. Whichever form of the pose you choose, it is all good for improving your ability to balance. Breathe here for about five breath cycles. Bring your foot back to the floor. Try Tree Pose standing on your other leg. Notice the difference from one side to the other. Observe how you feel now.

TRAUMA-INFORMED AND TRAUMA-RESPONSIVE YOGA TEACHING

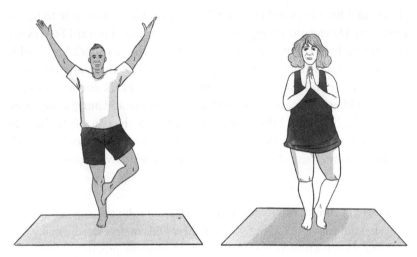

FIGURE 17.1A AND FIGURE 17.1B TREE POSE

2. ALTERNATE NOSTRIL BREATHING (*NADI SHODHANAM*)

Alternate nostril breathing is generally a calming practice, but there are always outliers who find the practice energizing. For this reason, it is a good idea to practice this first, so you know how it affects you. This breath can be taught to children as young as five and to people in their 90s. Feel free to make it your go-to practice for preparing for sleep (and for getting back to sleep in the middle of the night). The mind gets quiet when it is encouraged to focus on one thing and one thing only.

Begin in Easy Sitting Pose or Chair Mountain (or even in Corpse Pose). Sit with your spine straight. Notice how you are feeling. Put the index and middle fingers of your right hand together. Place the tips of these two fingers against the skin between your eyebrows. As you do this, you will notice that your ring finger and thumb are in a position to close one nostril at a time as in Figure 17.2.

Begin by closing the left nostril with the ring finger. Inhale through the right nostril for a count of three. Pause. Release the left nostril, and close the right nostril with the thumb. Exhale through the left nostril for a count of three. Inhale through the left nostril for a count of three. Pause. Release the right nostril and close the left nostril with the ring finger. Exhale through the right nostril for a count of three. Pause. Repeat three more times alternating sides (inhale right, exhale left, inhale left, exhale right). Check in with yourself. Notice the effect on your nervous system.

PRACTICES THAT BALANCE AND INTEGRATE

Quick Variation: Simply close the right nostril and breathe only through the left nostril for several minutes. This practice is generally very calming.

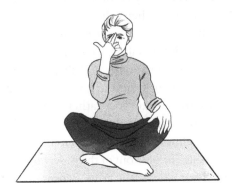

FIGURE 17.2 ALTERNATE NOSTRIL BREATHING

3. SPINAL EXTENSION POSE

Spinal Extension Pose is a balancing and strengthening pose that elongates the spine.

Begin on all fours on your mat. Raise your left arm in front of you and your right leg behind you. Go for length rather than height, keeping your arm and leg in line with or below your spine as in Figure 17.3a. Balance here. Find your breath. Come back to all fours. Repeat on the other side. Move from one side to the other for five repetitions on each side. Rest in Child's Pose. Notice any difference between each side.

Variation: Begin on all fours. Take your right hand towards the top of your mat and let it rest on the mat. Extend your left foot back, resting your toes towards the back of your mat. From here raise your arm and leg in line with your spine (but not higher) and then let your arm and toes come back to the mat as in Figure 17.3b. Repeat this action five times on each side. Rest in Child's Pose.

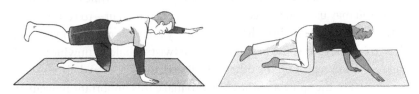

FIGURE 17.3A AND FIGURE 17.3B SPINAL EXTENSION POSE

4. WARRIOR POSE 3 (*VIRABHADRASANA 3*)

Warrior Pose 3 is a strong, grounding, and balancing pose. Begin in Mountain Pose, facing the short end of your mat. Step back with the left foot three to four feet. Inhale to prepare, then exhale as you tip your weight onto the front (right) foot at the same time as you are lifting your back (left) foot off the floor, heel first towards the ceiling. Pause. Inhale and find your balance on the right foot and place your arms in a "T" shape as in Figure 17.4a, gazing towards the floor (like a plane). Keep your hips square to the floor if you can.

Think about the length of the pose rather than the height of your leg. Exhale. Stay here for three more breaths or take your hands straight out from your shoulders, palms facing each other as in Figure 17.4b. Pause and take three more breaths. To come out of the pose, inhale, then exhale, drop the back foot to the floor, release the arms. Repeat on the other side.

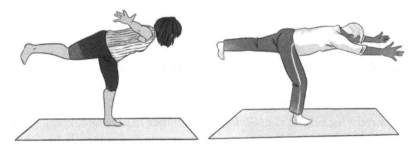

FIGURE 17.4A AND FIGURE 17.4B WARRIOR POSE 3

5. SEATED TWIST POSE (*PARIVRTTA SUKHASANA*)

Twists have long been a staple of yoga practice. Each twist has a gentle wringing effect on the spine.

There are many versions of twists. Here are four simple ones. Begin sitting in Chair Mountain Pose as in Figure 17.5a or in Easy Sitting Pose as in Figure 17.5b. Inhale to prepare and lengthen through the torso, then begin to twist to one side on your exhale. When you have fully exhaled, pause and find a natural breath in and out through the nose while staying in the twist. You may use your arms—or the arms of your chair—to rest on while in the twist for several breaths. Do not use your arms or the arms of your chair to crank your spine beyond a simple twist. Inhale to unwind; exhale and rest. Then repeat on the other side. Practice often, even daily, to keep a suppleness to the spine and the ability to make this important movement.

PRACTICES THAT BALANCE AND INTEGRATE

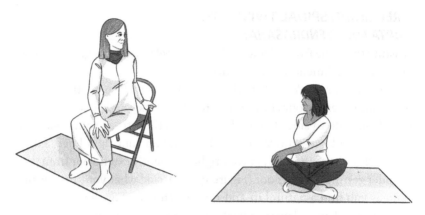

FIGURE 17.5A AND FIGURE 17.5B SEATED TWIST POSE

6. ALTERNATIVE SEATED TWIST POSE (*BHARADVAJA'S TWIST*)

This twist begins in Staff Pose. Bend the knees to one side. As you inhale, lengthen through the spine to prepare, then exhale and twist to one side, going only as far as your natural exhalation allows as in Figure 17.6. Pause. Breathe; let your head and neck follow the twist naturally. Breathe here for up to a minute. You may use your arms to support the twist. When twisting right, let the left hand rest on the right thigh and the right hand behind your back on the mat. Keep your torso upright as you twist. Exhale to unwind and rest. Repeat on the other side. Notice the difference on each side.

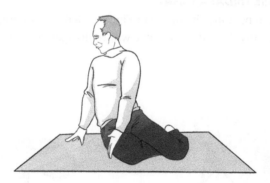

FIGURE 17.6 ALTERNATIVE SEATED TWIST POSE

7. RECLINING SPINAL TWIST POSE (*SUPTA MATSYENDRASANA*)

Twisting the spine from a lying position can feel rejuvenating. Let yourself enjoy the refreshment of this practice.

Begin in Corpse Pose. Bend the knees. Inhale to prepare, then exhale, draw your knees to your chest (Knees to Chest Pose), and gently rock your spine from side to side. Then inhale, extend the left leg to the mat and keep the right knee bent. With your left hand on your right knee, exhale and gently twist to the left. Let your right arm gently extend out from your shoulder resting on the floor (Figure 17.7). Decide what your neck wants to do as you find a natural in-and-out breath here. Stay here for five to seven breaths. Unwind on your next exhale. Inhale, then exhale as you draw both knees into the chest. Repeat on the other side. Notice the difference between each side as you rest in Corpse Pose.

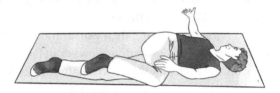

FIGURE 17.7 RECLINING SPINAL TWIST POSE

8. CAT POSE (*BIDALASANA*)

This pose can be done sitting (as in Figure 17.8a) or standing and is often paired with Cow Pose. It is a reliable way to dissipate tension in the spine.

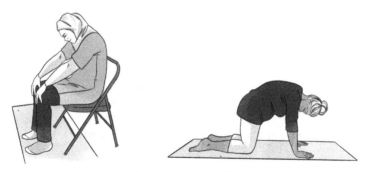

FIGURE 17.8A AND FIGURE 17.8B CAT POSE

Begin on all fours on your mat, hands under your shoulders, feet hip-width apart as in Figure 17.8b. This position is also called neutral spine or Table

PRACTICES THAT BALANCE AND INTEGRATE

Top. Notice your breath. Now, start to move your spine, exploring the movement beginning at the tailbone. Round your spine. Really notice how this feels. Breathe into this roundedness for a few breaths. Then explore the sensation as you return to a neutral spine.

9. COW POSE (*BITILASANA*)

This pose can be done sitting (as in Figure 17.9a) or standing and is often paired with Cat Pose. It is also a reliable way to dissipate tension in the spine.

Begin on all fours on your mat, hands under your shoulders, feet hip-width apart as in Figure 17.9b. Notice your breath. Inhale and begin to lift your chest. Notice if your spine feels compression in the low back. If it does, do less. Exhale. Breathe a natural in-and-out breath here and feel the shape of the pose. Exhale to release. Return to a neutral spine.

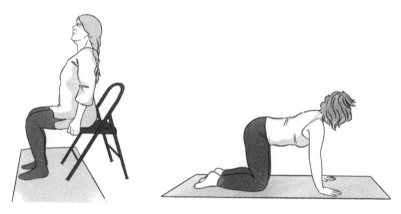

FIGURE 17.9A AND FIGURE 17.9B COW POSE

PIGEON: THREE VARIATIONS (*KAPOTASANA*)

Pigeon Pose allows you to externally rotate one hip at a time, an important action missing from regular standing and sitting activities. Many people are not particularly aware of their hips, but functional hip mobility is essential to many daily activities, such as getting dressed and moving around. Therefore, rotating your hips is certainly a helpful action to assist you in putting your pants on in the morning. Keeping your ball-and-socket joint mobile may be good for your emotional health too.

Pigeon Pose can be done from the floor, sitting, or lying on your back. In knowing all three variations, you can better accommodate your students' differing needs and body types. You do not need to feel sensation in this pose for there to be benefit. If you have tight hips, you may feel sensation. If you have more mobility in your hips, you may not feel sensation. But either way, external rotation is happening.

10. SEATED PIGEON POSE (*KAPOTASANA*)

Begin in Chair Mountain. Lift your right ankle and rest it on your left knee as in Figure 17.10. If it doesn't want to go there easily, let your right foot rest on your left shin. Put your right hand on your right knee and gently guide your knee slightly toward the floor. Don't force the movement. Take five natural breaths here. Uncross your leg. Pause. Repeat on the other side. Notice if one side was easier than the other.

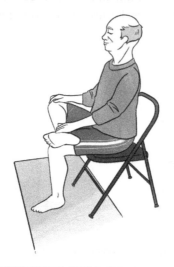

FIGURE 17.10 SEATED PIGEON POSE

11. PIGEON POSE ON THE MAT

Start on all fours on your mat. Inhale and take your left knee forward while rotating your hip to the left. Exhale and find a landing spot as the side of your left leg rests on the mat. Find a natural breath here while supporting your body weight with your hands under your shoulders. If you feel ease here, lower down to your forearms, bending your elbows as in Figure 17.11. If you feel at ease here, feel free to lower your head to the mat or place a block under your head for support. Continue breathing here for about a minute or so. This is a pose of surrender. Be aware of tension or gripping in your hip. Try to release any tension you are aware of. Allow the face to soften and your jaw to relax. Stay here for ten breath cycles or longer if you have time. Slowly reverse out of the pose and return to all fours. Rest in Child's Pose for three breaths. Repeat on the other side.

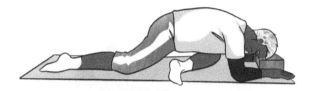

FIGURE 17.11 PIGEON POSE ON THE MAT

12. RECLINING PIGEON POSE

Begin in Corpse Pose. Bend your knees with your feet on the mat. Place your right foot on your left thigh near the knee. If this feels comfortable, take your right hand and push your right knee gently away from your body as in Figure 17.12. Breathe a natural breath for three breaths. Release your hand; rest your legs and let them extend. Repeat on the other side. Again, notice if there is a difference between your left and right sides.

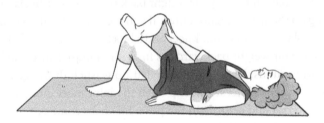

FIGURE 17.12 RECLINING PIGEON POSE

13. STAFF POSE (*DANDASANA*)

Staff Pose looks fairly basic—sitting with your legs straight out in front of you with a tall spine—yet it can take a lot of effort to find ease here. It is very helpful for postural awareness. Using a folded blanket underneath the tailbone like a wedge can be helpful.

Begin in Easy Sitting Pose. Lengthen through the spine and stretch your legs out in front of you. Hips are under the shoulders. Heels are in line with the hips. Inhale and draw your belly button towards your spine to gently engage your abdominal muscles. Exhale while still engaging the abdominal muscles as in Figure 17.13. Breathe in and out for three more breaths. If your hamstrings are really tight, place blocks or a rolled-up blanket under your knees.

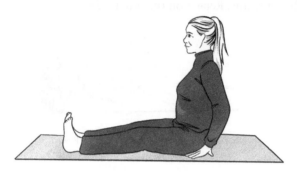

17.13 STAFF POSE

14. HERO POSE (*VIRASANA*)

Hero Pose is great for improving your posture and stretching the knees, ankles, and thighs. If you have had recent knee or hip injuries, props can be helpful.

Begin on all fours on your mat. Move into a kneeling position. Inhale and gently exhale, moving your weight back towards your heels until you are sitting on them as in Figure 17.14a. If you are unable to sit on your heels, try using a blanket under your knees and a block on its highest end to sit on as you take your weight backwards as in Figure 17.14b. Pause and breathe here for five rounds. Lastly, a small rolled-up washcloth wedged into the back of one or both knees will help open the joint more comfortably and allow you to rest and breathe in the pose. Inhale to come out of the pose. Exhale and rest in Child's Pose.

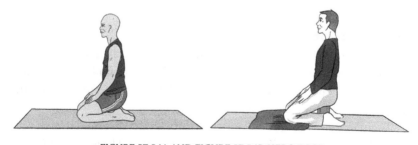

FIGURE 17.14A AND FIGURE 17.14B HERO POSE

PRACTICES THAT BALANCE AND INTEGRATE

15. DANCER POSE (*NATARAJASANA*)

Dancer Pose opens the chest and improves balance and strength.

Begin in Mountain Pose. Inhale and shift your weight to your right foot. Then reach your left hand behind you to your left foot as you bend your left knee and grab your foot from the inside of the ankle. The right leg is strong and straight. Draw your heel in toward your buttocks. Find your breath. Raise your right hand with your palm facing up as you lean forward into the pose hinging at the hip as in Figure 17.15. Stay here for three full breath cycles. Return to Mountain Pose. If you are struggling to balance or hold your foot steady, use the wall for support. Notice if you can find ease in the pose when you let your lifted hand rest on the wall or a chair back.

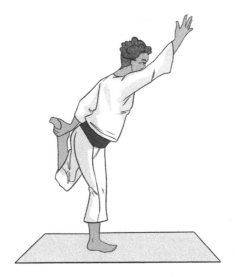

FIGURE 17.15 DANCER POSE

16. EAGLE POSE (*GARUDASANA*)

Eagle Pose can seem a little daunting at first. It can help with shoulder strain, while also improving balance. It has the added benefit of crossing the midline of the body, which may stimulate both hemispheres of the brain. This pose can also be done sitting in a chair with the wrists and ankles crossed.

Begin in Mountain Pose. Cross the left foot in front of the right foot, letting the left toes rest on the ground. Find your balance here. If your breath is steady, lift the left leg, bending at the knee, and cross it further over your right leg. At the same time, bend the right knee slightly. Keep your hips square to the front of your mat. With both knees bent, hug your legs toward each other. Start with your arms in a "T" and inhale, then swoop your arms inwards until your elbows connect—left arm under the right arm. As your elbows bend, let the backs of your palms move towards each other until they touch. Lift your elbows as in Figure 17.16a. Balance here for five breaths.

Alternatively, for the upper-body part of this pose, begin with your wrists crossed, palms toward the floor. Rotate your palms inward until the fingers interlace. Then, draw the interlaced hands in and up to rest at your chest. Simply cross the ankles instead of the whole leg and keep both feet on the mat as in Figure 17.16b. Breathe here for five breaths. Uncross and unwind. Notice how you feel.

If you find yourself struggling with this pose, keep it light. I (JS) can remember laughing so hard that it was impossible to balance. Let it be okay that not all poses make sense to your body when you first try them. All I could think was "I had no idea that restraining myself from peeing was a yoga pose."

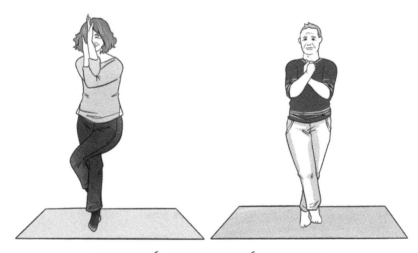

FIGURE 17.16A AND FIGURE 17.16B EAGLE POSE

17. LATERAL SPINE MOVEMENT

Lateral Spine Movement is moving the spine laterally or simply from side to side. It can easily be done standing or sitting in a chair. In a group setting, you may need to coordinate the movement if you are using the extended arm version—that is, have everyone move the same way at the same time. It is nearly always a "feel good" pose that elevates your mood.

Begin in Mountain Pose or Chair Mountain.

Sitting or standing, the spine is straight, the chest lifted slightly. Let

PRACTICES THAT BALANCE AND INTEGRATE

your hands rest on your hips. Inhale to prepare, then exhale and lean your whole body to the left as in Figure 17.17. Inhale and return to center. Repeat on the other side. Feel free to experiment with where you place your arms. Try them with your fingers on your shoulders. Or, as a longer lever, reach one hand to the ceiling and one hand towards the floor. Notice which one feels better for your spine today. Repeat several times on each side.

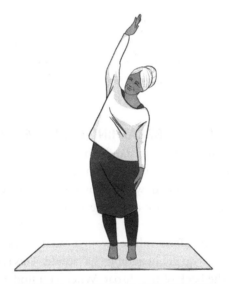

FIGURE 17.17 LATERAL SPINE MOVEMENT

18. BALANCING HALF MOON POSE (*ARDHA CHANDRASANA*)

Balancing Half Moon Pose is a great asymmetrical balancing pose that helps build strength and focus. Begin in Mountain Pose at the top of your mat. Step your right foot back three to four feet similar to the Warrior Pose 2 set-up. Choose your prop: a chair, window ledge, etc. as in Figure 17.18a or a block as in Figure 17.18b. Let the left knee bend as you reach down to the floor or your prop. When your hand is firmly in place, let the right leg rise, straight back with your foot flexed. Your left leg is straight, your knee soft. Find your breath here. When you feel stable, take your right hand towards the ceiling and start to revolve your torso. If your balance is steady, let your gaze follow your hand to the ceiling.

If you feel unstable, look straight ahead or continue looking at the floor. Find a natural breath here and balance for five breaths. Unwind and rest in Mountain Pose. Repeat on the other side. Compare the difference from one side to the other. Another fun way to practice this pose is against a wall.

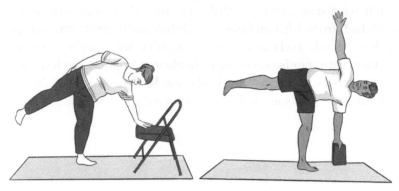

FIGURE 17.18A AND FIGURE 17.18B BALANCING HALF MOON POSE

19. OCEAN-SOUNDING BREATHING (*UJJAYI PRANAYAMA*)

Ocean-Sounding Breathing, as a stand-alone practice, can be done sitting either at the beginning of class to tune in and allow you to focus, or as a resting practice as you wind down your practice. It can both help activate the parasympathetic response of the nervous system and build heat in the body.

Begin in Easy Sitting Pose. Inhale through your nose and exhale through your mouth making a quiet but audible "ha" sound. This is the constriction of the glottis at the back of the throat. When you find a rhythm to your breath, close your lips and still make the same "ha" sound. Do this for two to three minutes. Notice how you feel.

20. MEDITATION

This short meditation explores what it feels like to create a foundation for joy. True joy comes from a foundation, steadiness, and a ventral-vagal-state kind of knowing that you are safe and it is okay to allow joy. Find a comfortable seated position with your back straight. Feel free to have your eyes open or closed. If they are closed, gaze at the back of your eyelids if you want. It is often easier to do this practice with your eyes closed. If closing your eyes is not comfortable for you today, simply soften your gaze.

Notice your connection to the ground or chair below you. Engage in an active pressing down of your feet or legs and your sitting bones. From the sensations or pressing down, draw up through the center of your core, through your belly, heart, and up through the crown of your head. Simultaneously, soften your shoulders, your jaw, and the muscles around your eyes. Invite in a half-smile, gently drawing the corners of your mouth toward the

PRACTICES THAT BALANCE AND INTEGRATE

outside edge of your eyes. If you'd like, place your hands on your heart. You might say to yourself, "I am grounded, balanced, and supported."

Bringing your hands to your side, perhaps supporting yourself with the floor or the arms of your chair, shift your weight to the right. Notice any change in your breath, your muscles, and your sense of balance. Breathe and hold this shift for four or five extended breaths. Come back to your center. Once you are back to center, notice your breath, your muscles, and your sense of balance. Press down and lift up again. Pause and bring your hands to your heart. If you lost your half-smile, find it. You might say to yourself, "I am grounded, balanced, and supported."

In the same way, supporting yourself with your hands, shift to the left side. Notice any change in your breath, your muscles, and your sense of balance. Breathe and hold this shift for four or five extended breaths. Come back to center. Once you are back to center, notice your breath, your muscles, and your sense of balance. Press down and lift up. Pause and bring your hands to your heart and remember your half-smile. You might say to yourself, "I am grounded, balanced, and supported."

Now, pressing down and lifting up in an integrated way, allow your breath to move naturally in and out. Notice your half-smile. You might say to yourself, "I am grounded, balanced, and supported." Now, ask yourself, your body, "What if there was joy?" Place your hands on your heart and ask your body again, "What if there was joy?" Allow any sensations you may notice. Notice their location, shape, energy, direction (up, radiating out). Notice what action urges might be there for your smile to grow, your heart to lift up, an openness. Allow for whatever comes up. Perhaps it is a protection, closing. Perhaps there is an absence of sensation. Allow what is.

When you are ready, notice your breath and your sense of balance. Orient toward your half-smile. Say to yourself, "I am grounded, balanced, and supported." Slowly open or raise your eyes and bring your awareness back to the room.

> **Journal Prompt.** Describe your relationship with balance, integration, and joy. For those who have been through trauma, the openness and lightness of joy can sometimes be scary or anxiety-provoking. How might it help to center a joy practice within the context of groundedness and balance? How might this work for other poses and practices you teach?

TEACHER TRAINING DISCUSSION QUESTIONS

1. Name three poses in English and in Sanskrit that can balance the nervous system.

2. Name elements of each of the three poses that contribute to the balancing effect.

3. Should balancing practices be part of every yoga class? Why or why not?

4. What are two simple ways to modify a balancing or integrating pose?

5. How might balance and integration create a foundation for joy?

CHAPTER 18

Cultivating a Trauma-Informed and Responsive Yoga Space

prâtibhâd vâ sarvam

Yoga Sutra III:34

By perfectly concentrated Meditation on the heart, the interior being, comes the knowledge of consciousness [knowing of the mind].

Charles Johnston (1912)

A trauma-informed and responsive (TIR) yoga space is something you cultivate over time. To do this well, you must acknowledge that physical and social environments can affect mood, attitude, behavior, physiological and emotional states, the experience of identity, and a person's feeling of worth and dignity, and can either inhibit or facilitate empowerment (Gill, 2019). The yoga space should be intentionally designed to facilitate growth and healing, reduce risk of harm or traumatization, and follow the basic principles of trauma-informed care (Butler *et al.*, 2011; Fallot & Harris, 2009; Gill, 2019):

Safety	Trustworthiness and Transparency
Peer Support	Collaboration and Mutuality
Empowerment	Voice
Choice	Addresses Cultural, Historical, and Gender Issues

The process of cultivating a TIR yoga space includes the consideration of everything from the yoga props and supports available in the studio to the development and support of the community. It includes careful thought and development of the physical, psychological, and social aspects of the space you are nurturing. In this chapter, we cover the considerations you might apply to your space so that it is trauma-informed and responsive.

Disclaimer: We Can't Promise a Safe Space

Offering a *safe space* is not possible. Feeling safe is a subjective experience and, as such, cannot be assured. Given various experiences and identities, there can be no universal experience of safety. No matter how determined you are, there is no way that risk can be completely eliminated, especially when there is an inherent imbalance of power and privilege (Roze des Ordons *et al.*, 2022).

> **TIR PRINCIPLE:** YOU CANNOT PROMISE A SAFE SPACE
> Offering a safe space is not possible. Feeling safe is a subjective experience and, as such, cannot be assured.

Some use the term *brave space* to acknowledge the infeasibility of safety and emphasize the courage required to engage in difficult and honest dialogue (Roze des Ordons *et al.*, 2022). This approach, however, often places the burden of being courageous on marginalized and underrepresented students (Roze des Ordons *et al.*, 2022). Others use the term *accountable spaces* to emphasize the shared responsibility in creating an inclusive and welcoming environment and to work toward alignment between what is intended and the impact that language and behavior yield (Roze des Ordons *et al.*, 2022). Although this is better, it fails to recognize how students' diversity, identities, previous experiences (stress and trauma), and unique present-day challenges can influence their sense of personal safety. To do that, more trauma-informed and responsive spaces are needed.

You—It's Not All About the Space

Where you teach may change with time and opportunity. Perhaps you will teach in a lovely, clean, quiet, spacious space dedicated for yoga practice. Or you may be relegated to the back hallway in a school (we kid you not, it has happened)—dark and dusty, cramped, and smelly. Or maybe your spot is in the middle of a road, and you teach a pose every time the lights change—metaphorically speaking, of course. My (JS) yoga teaching has covered this gamut and has included busy street corners. The common denominator to your teaching space will be you and your nervous system.

> **TIR PRINCIPLE:** TIR YOGA TEACHERS SELF-REGULATE
> Take time to self-regulate as part of your personal and pre-teaching practices.

Deb Dana, author of *Polyvagal Theory in Therapy* (2018), says if there is only one person in the room in a ventral vagal state, it should be you! This is true for us as yoga teachers. The only way we know how to reliably access a ventral vagal state is through the daily practice of yoga and an abiding commitment to caring for self through nourishing food, getting enough fresh air, and guarding sleep routine, to name just a few daily practices—feel free to call them routines or habits—that sustain you for the long haul.

As you work to be a TIR yoga teacher, you are developing the capacity to sustainably embody connection states as you teach. This is important and comes from your relationship with your nervous system. As you embody connection states (i.e., rest, restoration, and recovery; alert engagement; and challenge and growth; see Table 18.1), you *communicate* a nonverbal sense of ease, acceptance, and loving-kindness to your students. It is in a self-regulated state of connection that the nervous system can most readily learn. Arriving at a yoga session or class in a self-regulated, connection state requires an ongoing awareness of your state of activation and corresponding practices to either move you to or center yourself in connection states.

Table 18.1 Trauma-Informed and Responsive Teaching and the Connection States

Connection States (Ventral Vagal States)		
State of Embodiment	What It Feels Like	Embodiment of Connection States while Teaching
Rest, Restoration, and Recovery	Safe and Relaxed	**Body:** soft, relaxed muscles, gentle stance **Breath:** smooth, even, subtle **Voice:** soft, soothing, gentle, warm, caring
Alert Engagement	Safe	**Body:** engaged, active, grounded, solid stance **Breath:** smooth, active diaphragm **Voice:** engaged, animated, balanced and strong

cont.

| Connection States (Ventral Vagal States) ||||
State of Embodiment	What It Feels Like	Embodiment of Connection States while Teaching
Challenge and Growth	Safe and Activated	**Body:** engaged, active, grounded, stable **Breath:** active, steady **Voice:** resonant, enthusiastic, effectively projected

> **Journal Prompt.** What are the practices and routines that you engage in to support your nervous system so that you can teach from a ventral vagal state? In what ways do you interact with students reinforcing a ventral vagal connection?

Even with the best of intentions, life can get in the way of class preparation time. Consider the mantra "presence over perfection." Consider what you might do when the supports you have in place to prepare for class fall apart. Do you cancel? Quickly sub out? What are the consequences of your choices? What does this do for your work toward being reliable and trustworthy? Can we both manage life and its inherent unpredictability and show up for class self-regulated, grounded, and ready to teach from a state of connection? Consider the experience of these two teachers.

> Every teacher has a different way of preparing to teach. There are many variations of pre-teaching preparations. For one stark contrast, consider Sonja (she/her), yoga teacher and mother of two toddlers who lived walking distance to the studio. The other, Rachel (she/her), a yoga teacher who worked part-time, taught yoga part-time, and lived a 30-minute drive from the studio. Sonja, the mother of two, said she had to drive over even though the walk would have been good for her and a sound way to prepare for class. However, the babysitter often did not arrive in enough time to allow for walking. She explained her best effort was to park at the back door, sigh deeply as she got out of her car, and take deep belly breaths as she walked up the steps and down the long hallway to the studio. She would say, "This is what I have to offer today. May it be enough." And it was. In contrast, Rachel, the other yoga teacher, once called the manager of the studio in a "flap" to help her find a sub for her evening class; her reason was that she had to work a bit later than she thought and she wouldn't have the usual hour she needed to prepare herself for class.

Neither of these methods or timing for preparation to teach a class is right or wrong. But they do give an example of the spectrum from the ideal to the practical and sense of "this is the best I can do today" that you may experience yourself. The point is that you do intentionally make time to prepare yourself and have a good handle on what it takes for you to teach a good class.

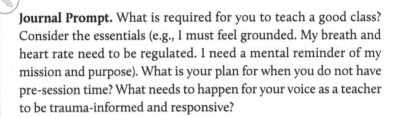

Journal Prompt. What is required for you to teach a good class? Consider the essentials (e.g., I must feel grounded. My breath and heart rate need to be regulated. I need a mental reminder of my mission and purpose). What is your plan for when you do not have pre-session time? What needs to happen for your voice as a teacher to be trauma-informed and responsive?

Community of Care

Gail Parker reminds us what it means to be part of a yoga community inclusive in the sense of connection, shared needs, and common goals:

> Community is not a location, an organization, or a place where people gather. Community is a sense of connection and relationship among people with shared needs, interests, and common goals, designed to meet the common needs of the community members. (Parker, 2020, p. 143)

Wherever you teach, you will have the opportunity to create a TIR community that recognizes trauma as an important factor impacting health and wellbeing throughout a person's lifespan (Gill, 2019). In a TIR community, you balance the importance of acknowledging and celebrating the diverse range of personal identity and promoting voice and choice with the safety and wellbeing of the community (Gill, 2019). It is a practice of collective care within which both *me* and *we* matter.

> **TIR PRINCIPLE:** CULTIVATE COMMUNITIES OF CARE
> TIR communities are continuously developing and evolving communities of care.

We, the authors, do not need to develop an extensive list of practices for how to guide community behavior. Patanjali's *Yoga Sutras* provides the eight limbs of yoga as a path to purposeful and conscious living (Parker, 2020). The paths were designed to work hierarchically. That means the first two limbs—Yama and Niyama—provide a foundation for the rest (Parker, 2020). Dr. Gail Parker asserts that these ten practices can be the foundation of conscious communities of care and connection. The Yamas guide us in how we relate to others and our world—ahimsa (non-harming), satya (truth), asteya (non-stealing), brahmacharya (moderation), and aparigraha (non-attachment) (Parker, 2020; Ranganathan, 2008). The Niyamas guide us in our inner observances—saucha (purity), tapas (inner heat), santosha (contentment), svadhyaya (self-study), and ishvara pranidhana (surrender to your higher power) (Parker, 2020; Ranganathan, 2008). See Dr. Parker's (2020) book, *Restorative Yoga for Ethnic and Race-Based Stress and Trauma*, for a detailed exploration of how the Yamas and Niyamas help support community.

> **TIR PRINCIPLE:** YOGA OFFERS GUIDANCE
> TIR communities study and practice the Yamas and Niyamas.

The four immeasurables, also from Patanjali's *Yoga Sutras*, further guide us in the nature of how we can relate to ourselves and others. Clearly qualities of ventral vagal connection states—equanimity, compassion, joy, and loving-kindness—remind us that we are always in relationship and that the nature of our actions is central to the quality of those relationships (Goddard, 2021). If we are truly committed to these practices, we would have our community of care. I (CCC) once attended a gathering in which yoga teachers and community leaders from all over the world were discussing and debating diversity, inclusion, equity, and TIR practice. Over and over, we kept coming back to the teachings of Patanjali's *Yoga Sutras* as our guide.

> **TIR PRINCIPLE:** CREATE COMMUNITY AGREEMENTS
> Community agreements can support TIR practices.

TIR PRACTICE: COMMUNITY AGREEMENTS

It can be helpful to develop and share community agreements during trainings, gatherings, and group experiences. They are best when they manifest from the group and are tailored to the group's needs and preferences. Community agreements help support several of the basic principles of trauma-informed care—transparency, safety, voice, and collaboration. Below is a list of agreements to consider (listed alphabetically in order not to inadvertently elevate any one value or practice):

- Agency—acknowledge each person's right to be self-determined.
- Amplify—the voices of those at the margins.
- Be trauma-informed and responsive—use TIR tools to support your interactions with yourself and others.
- Challenge—ideas and behaviors, not the person.
- Compassion—remembering that we are all trying and won't always get it right.
- Confidentiality—honor each person's right to privacy; consider when something is not your story to tell.
- Connection—take the time to ground, breathe, and then engage from a ventral vagal connection state.
- Consent—secure ongoing, informed consent (for touch, personal inquiries, intense content).
- Diversity—respect each person's identity, context, and community.
- Identity—recognize your own and others' identity(ies) and don't assume the identity of others. Share and use correct names, pronunciations, and pronouns.
- Learning—center learning and growth, not agreement, closure, and perfection.
- Listening—practice mindful and heartful listening.
- Name—gently and with compassion name the elephants in the room.
- Nonviolence—practice nonviolent communication.
- Positionality—be mindful of your privileges and identities.
- Respect—be respectful in voice and actions.
- Safety—prioritize the safety of each member of the community.
- Share—from your own experience using "I" statements.
- Silence—honor silence and time for reflection.
- Space—create space for multiple truths, voices, and experiences.
- Understanding—acknowledge intent and address impact. Call in, not out.

> **TIR PRINCIPLE:** OFFER YOGA AS A SPIRITUAL AND SECULAR PRACTICE
> TIR yoga honors the spirituality of yoga while providing practices that are welcoming to all.

TIR PRACTICE: YOGA AS A SPIRITUAL AND SECULAR PRACTICE

Yoga is a spiritual practice. Many, including the two authors of this book, describe the transformational effect that yoga has had in their lives. This is spiritual—the shifting of our inner worlds, a transformative change (Cook-Cottone *et al.*, 2019). Something can be spiritual and secular. *Secularity* means not pertaining to, or connecting with, a specific religion. Rather than promoting a position of non-belief, a secular approach invites you to bring your own belief system into the learning experience (Cook-Cottone *et al.*, 2019). This is a very important and critical point. How can you cultivate a yoga space that will feel inviting and inclusive to someone who is Jewish, Christian, Buddhist, Muslim, or of any other religious practice?

> **TIR PRINCIPLE:** TRAUMA-INFORMED AND RESPONSIVE SPACES ARE UNIQUE
> TIR spaces are developed and maintained to meet the unique histories, needs, and preferences of the community.

TIR PRACTICE: CREATING A TRAUMA-INFORMED AND RESPONSIVE SPACE

As with TIR teaching, cultivating your TIR space will be a process of attuning to your students, their identities and intersectionality, and what will be most effective in supporting their nervous systems. This will look different from space to space, because each community presents its own set of histories, needs, and preferences. Table 18.2 includes the aspects of your space and possible considerations. This is not an exhaustive list of considerations. Examples are provided in each section to ignite and help shape discussion.

CULTIVATING A TRAUMA-INFORMED AND RESPONSIVE YOGA SPACE

Table 18.2 Considerations for Creating a TIR Space

Yoga	• Yoga centers on appreciation of, and connection to, the body and development of the self. • The focus is on the journey and process rather than the perfect expression of a pose, practice, form, or outcome. • Practice and teaching is done with a spirit of inquiry and exploration, rather than fixing, correcting, and idealism. • All eight limbs of yoga are taught and practiced, and there is instruction in key concepts such as impermanence (sensations and all things arise and pass), suffering (attachment and aversion), and not self (development of self as witness). • Yoga philosophy and history is honored and shared as an integrated part of yoga teaching and practice. • Yoga symbols, Sanskrit, and artifacts are only used in historical and philosophical contexts. • Yoga is taught and practiced using a TIR approach. • Yoga is taught in a spiritual and philosophical yet secular manner. • There are regular opportunities for continuing education in topics associated with TIR teaching, accessibility, yoga philosophy, positive embodiment, and methods for teaching all eight limbs of yoga. • Community members consistently seek to know and understand yoga philosophy, practices, and history. • See the Accessible Yoga Association's *The Love of Yoga Podcast* with Anjali Rao (www.accessibleyoga.org/podcasts/the-love-of-yoga) for regular podcasts on the teachings of yoga.
Teachers	• Teachers seek to embody mindful awareness, being with and working with skills, and the yoga and mindful self-care practices they desire for their students. • Teachers actively engage in practices that help them be self-regulated and able to be present in a ventral vagal connection state for their students. • Teachers are diverse in age, body shapes, gender identity, ethnicity and race, sexual orientation, and backgrounds. • Teachers are trained in TIR yoga teaching, diversity equity, inclusion, and accessibility. • Teachers do not engage in negative body-talk in any form (e.g., comments on weight, body parts, shape, diets). • Yoga teachers adhere to yoga ethical guidelines. • Teachers work within their scope of practice. • Teachers seek support and care when they are struggling. • Teachers feel valued, supported, and respected.

cont.

Safety	- There are at least two clearly marked, accessible exits.
- The studio has a first-aid kit.
- Nonjudgmentally, in private settings, community members check in on those who appear at risk (e.g., "I noticed x, y, z, and I wanted to make sure you are okay. I have been worried about you. Are you okay?").
- There is a referral database for local specialists in fields such as physical therapy, nutrition, and mental health support.
- There is a defibrillator and members of staff are trained on how to use it.
- Teachers are trained in cardiopulmonary resuscitation (CPR).
- Waivers and acknowledgment of primary care physician approval of practice are secured.
- There is signage relevant to safety and safety regulations.
- There is no use of alcohol or other substances associated with yoga and yoga practices (e.g., this is a sober space).
- All teachers, administration/management, and staff work within their scope of practice.
Props	- There are supports such as having plain, metal folding chairs on hand for accommodating varied body types and abilities.
- Props are easy to access and modeled by yoga teachers.
- Using props is normalized (e.g., props are frequently utilized with students at all ability levels).
- There are enough props for everyone.
- See Chapter 15 for a list of recommended props.
Privacy	- There is visual privacy (e.g., people outside the room can't see in, like a storefront).
- There is sound privacy (e.g., you can't hear conversations in the adjoining room).
- There are private changing rooms or spaces.
- There are private places to have difficult conversations.
- There are suggestion, concern, and feedback boxes that can be used anonymously.
- Teachers, administration/management, and staff do not discuss students outside of private conversations related to organization, business, and safety/wellbeing concerns.

Physical Space	- The physical space promotes a sense of safety, soothing, and calmness.
- The occupancy guides ensure there is sufficient space for each student.
- The mats can be set in a circle or semi-circle so no one is behind someone else.
- There is plenty of space to practice near a wall or with a wall behind you.
- The rest rooms are far enough away for privacy and not so far that there is a sense of isolation or being alone to get to them.
- There are locks on the bathroom and changing-room doors.
Music	- Music is respectful to all identities and bodies.
- Music supports, not drives, the yoga experience.
- Consider using instrumental music or not using music at all.
Merchandise	- Clothing is available in a variety of sizes and ranges of coverage for the body.
- If books are sold, texts include traditional texts, texts on accessibility, and texts on the history of yoga.
- There are no products being sold that support risky or unhealthy behaviors (e.g., cleanses and dietary aids that have not been medically vetted).
Medical and Nutritional Advice	- Teachers, administration/management, and staff work within their scope of practice and refer to community specialists when needed.
- Teachers do not undermine students' relationships with their therapists, doctors, or nutritionists.
- Nutritional guidance, if offered, is provided by a licensed dietitian or nutritionist.
- Warning signs for eating disorders, excessive exercise, addiction, and other mental health issues are posted with guidance for how to secure support.
- Information sheets are available providing useful referrals for expert nutritional supports, mental health assessment and treatment, physical therapy, and medical support for injury.
Location and Access	- The location of your class is accessible for all bodies.
- There is adequate, accessible parking.
- The space is accessible by public transportation.
- If there are stairs, there is also an elevator.

cont.

Lighting	• Lights are soft (not harsh). • There are no shadows (can activate protective states). • Natural light is prioritized. • There are no dark corners or places in which you cannot see clearly enough to assess safety.
Decor	• There are signs, prints, and posters that remind students that all are welcome. • There are no signs and symbols in the space that have been appropriated from Indian culture or that lack context. • There are no mirrors, or you can orient away from or cover mirrors. • Wall art is conducive to all people feeling welcome. • Walls are painted in colors or patterns that have a more calming effect. • When possible, add plants. Plants, other nature-based decor, can be calming, improve mood, and increase a sense of connectedness to nature. • Arrangement of decorative objects creates more space, adds symmetry, and decreases a sense of crowding.
Cleanliness	• There are clear protocols for sweeping and mopping the floor. • There are clear protocols for cleaning mats and other props after they are used. • The studio or space meets all cleanliness guidelines and regulations. • Adherence to cleanliness protocols is a daily practice.
Boundaries	• Role boundaries are clear (administration/management, teachers, students). • Teachers set and maintain clear boundaries between themselves and their students. • There is a safe and clear way for students and teachers to communicate needs and seek support if they are struggling. • Yoga teachers not trained in TIR practices, inclusion, or accessibility are not permitted to teach classes. • There are organizational guidelines or codes defining boundaries and related behaviors. • The community does not encourage or celebrate over-exercise, pushing too hard in a pose practice, practicing to injury, excessive fasting or food restriction, and other behaviors that create a health risk.

Agency and Opting Out	• Students are encouraged to notice external and internal body sensations and use this information to make choices for and with their bodies. • Teachers encourage students to listen to their body cues with curiosity, such as: "Am I tired?"; "Does that hurt?"; "Does this feel good in my body?" • Teachers offer clear ways to accommodate, add support, and opt out of activities, hands-on assists, and other components of the class. • Options *always* include opting out. • There is ongoing permission for students to choose alternative versions of yoga poses and practices and to take breaks as needed.
Accessibility and Inclusion	• Options and accommodations are offered for each practice and pose. • The community engages in outreach that is specifically welcoming to and inclusive of a range of individuals. • The community prioritizes diversity and accessibility when hiring. • See the Accessible Yoga Association (www.accessibleyoga.org) for guidance and training. • See Dianne Bondy Yoga (www.diannebondyyoga.com) for training in accessibility, social justice, and equity. • See Michelle Cassandra Johnson (www.michellecjohnson.com) for training on yoga and social justice. • Read *My Grandmother's Hands: Racialized Trauma and the Pathway to Mending Our Hearts and Bodies* by Resmaa Menakem (www.resmaa.com)
Accountability	• There are clear pathways to report concerns and misconduct. • Students, teachers, and management/administration all have a voice in policy making. • Students, teachers, and management/administration are able to call for forums to discuss issues within the community. • Leaders welcome challenging ideas. • Administration/management reaches out to teachers about whom there are concerns, helps co-create plans for addressing issues, and monitors that the plans have been followed. • There is a board of directors, or a team to consult with, that consists of diverse members of the community including those in the field of mental health, medicine, individuals who represent key stakeholders in the community, and faculty or researchers if a university is in close proximity.

(Informed by Cook-Cottone, 2015, 2020, 2023; Cook-Cottone & Douglass, 2017; Gill, 2019; Parker, 2020)

TRAUMA-INFORMED AND TRAUMA-RESPONSIVE YOGA TEACHING

Journal Prompt. As you look over the list of variables to consider when developing and maintaining TIR space, what stands out for you? Why? What needs to happen for the place where you practice and teach to be more trauma-informed and responsive?

Closing

You have just finished the last chapter of this book. This chapter on creating a TIR yoga space is a wonderful place to close. In writing this book, both of the authors, Catherine and Joanne, have felt as if we are creating this book as a nurturing container, a space for you to learn and grow. It is our hope that the points of inquiry, the journaling, the science and the theory, and all of the practices have brought you a sense of confidence and empowerment as you go out into your communities to share yoga. You are ready now with effective and powerful tools for *being with* and *working with* what is present, in the right here and right now, including students in need of your support. You are ready to guide and empower your students.

It is a difficult process, the ending of something. This is where our yoga can help us again. In yoga, it is the endings that make space for the transformation into something new. So, thank you for learning and growing with us. We are so very honored to have been part of what is next for you!

TEACHER TRAINING DISCUSSION QUESTIONS

1. Give an example of a pre-teaching ritual. When are other times you might use this ritual? In what ways might this support your work?
2. Discuss the role of you, the teacher, in creating a TIR community space.
3. How might the Yamas and Niyamas help to support a community of care?
4. In what ways are community agreements helpful? In what contexts?
5. What does it mean to be both spiritual and secular? Explain the relationship to inclusion.
6. What would you add to the things to consider when developing and maintaining a TIR community space?

References

Aggarwal, A. K. (2020). *Gheranda Samhita: The Foundation of Modern Yoga*. Punjab, India: Devotees of Sri Sri Ravi Shanker Ashram.

American Medical Association (2021). Advancing Health Equity: A Guide to Language, Narrative, and Concepts. www.ama-assn.org/system/files/ama-aamc-equity-guide.pdf

American Psychiatric Association (2022). *Diagnostic and Statistical Manual of Mental Disorders: Diagnostic and Statistical Manual of Mental Disorders, Fifth Edition, Text Revision*. Arlington, VA: American Psychiatric Association.

American Psychological Association (2022). Inclusive language guidelines. www.apa.org/about/apa/equity-diversity-inclusion/language-guide.pdf

Ashwell, S. J., Baskin, P. K., Christiansen, S. L., DiBari, S. A., et al. (2023). Three recommended inclusive language guidelines for scholarly publishing: Words matter. *Learned Publishing, 36*(1), 94–99. https://doi.org/10.1002/leap.1527

Baitmangalkar, A. (2023). How can we work together to avoid cultural appropriation? Yoga International. https://yogainternational.com/article/view/how-we-can-work-together-to-avoid-cultural-appropriation-in-yoga

Barkataki, S. (2020). *Embrace Yoga's Roots: Courageous Ways to Deepen Your Yoga Practice*. Orlando, FL: Ignite Yoga and Wellness Institute.

Benjet, C., Bromet, E., Karam, E. G., Kessler, R. C., et al. (2016). The epidemiology of traumatic event exposure worldwide: Results from the World Mental Health Survey Consortium. *Psychological Medicine, 46*, 327–343.

Bohus, M., Dyer, A. S., Priebe, K., Krüger, A. et al. (2013). Dialectical behaviour therapy for post-traumatic stress disorder after childhood sexual abuse in patients with and without borderline personality disorder: A randomised controlled trial. *Psychotherapy and Psychosomatics, 82*(4), 221–233.

Butler, L. D., Critelli, F. M., & Rinfrette, E. S. (2011). Trauma-informed care and mental health. *Directions in Psychiatry, 31*, 197–210.

Bryce, I., Horwood, N., Cantrell, K., & Gildersleeve, J. (2022). Pulling the trigger: A systematic literature review of trigger warnings as a strategy for reducing traumatization in higher education. *Trauma, Violence & Abuse, 24*(4), 2882–2894.

Centers for Disease Control (2023a). Adverse Childhood Experiences (ACEs). www.cdc.gov/violenceprevention/aces/index.html

Centers for Disease Control (2023b). Fast facts: Preventing Adverse Childhood Experiences. www.cdc.gov/violenceprevention/aces/fastfact.html

Charles, A., Hare-Duke, L., Nudds, H., Franklin, D. et al. (2022). Typology of content warnings and trigger warnings: Systematic review. *PLoS ONE, 17*(5), e0266722. https://doi.org/10.1371/journal.pone.0266722

Church, D. (2019). *Emotional Freedom Technique: The EFT Manual*. Fulton, CA: Energy Psychology Press.

Clay, R. A. (2022). Are you experiencing compassion fatigue? American Psychological Association. www.apa.org/topics/covid-19/compassion-fatigue

Cook-Cottone, C. P. (2013). Dosage as a critical variable in yoga therapy research. *International Journal of Yoga Therapy, 23*(2), 11–12.

Cook-Cottone, C. P. (2015). *Mindfulness and Yoga: A Primer for Mental Health Professionals*. New York, NY: Springer.

Cook-Cottone, C. P. (2017). *Mindfulness and Yoga in Schools: A Guide for Teachers and Practitioners*. New York, NY: Springer.

Cook-Cottone, C. P. (2020). *Embodiment and the Treatment of Eating Disorders: The Body as a Resource in Recovery*. New York, NY: W. W. Norton.

Cook-Cottone, C. P. (2023). *The Embodied Healing Workbook: The Art and Science of Befriending Your Body in Trauma Recovery—Over 100 Healing Practices*. Eau Claire, WI: PESI.

Cook-Cottone, C. P., Childress, T., & Harper, J. C. (2019). Secularity: Guiding questions for inclusive yoga in schools. *International Journal of Yoga Therapy, 29*, 127–133.

Cook-Cottone, C. P., & Douglass, L. L. (2017). Yoga communities and eating disorders: Creating safe space for positive embodiment. *International Journal of Yoga Therapy, 27*(1), 87–93.

Cook-Cottone, C. P., & Guyker, W. M. (2018). The development and validation of the Mindful Self-Care Scale (MSCS): An assessment of practices that support positive embodiment. *Mindfulness, 9*, 161–175.

Cook-Cottone, C. P., LaVigne, M., Guyker, W., Travers, L., Lemish, E., & Elenson, P. (2017). Trauma-informed yoga: An embodied, cognitive-relational framework. *International Journal of Complementary and Alternative Medicine, 9*, 00284. http://dx.doi.org/10.15406/ijcam.2017.09.00284

Costa, P. L., McDuffie, J. W., Brown, S. E., He, Y. et al. (2023). Microaggressions: Mega problems or micro issues? A meta-analysis. *Journal of Community Psychology, 51*(1), 137–153.

Cramer, H., Anheyer, D., Saha, F. J., & Dobos, G. (2018). Yoga for posttraumatic stress disorder—a systematic review and meta-analysis. *BMC Psychiatry, 18*, 1–9.

Crenshaw, K. W. (2017). *On Intersectionality: Essential Writings*. New York, NY: The New Press.

Dana, D. (2018). *Polyvagal Theory in Therapy: Engaging the Rhythm of Regulation* (Norton Series on Interpersonal Neurobiology). New York, NY: W. W. Norton.

Dana, D. (2020). *Polyvagal Exercises for Safety and Connection: 50 Client-Centered Practices*. New York, NY: W. W. Norton.

REFERENCES

Desikachar, T. K. V. (1995). *The Heart of Yoga: Developing a Personal Practice.* Rochester, VT: Inner Traditions International.

Emerson, D. (2015). *Trauma-Sensitive Yoga in Therapy: Bringing the Body into Treatment.* New York, NY: W. W. Norton.

Emerson, D., & Hopper, E. (2011). *Overcoming Trauma Through Yoga: Reclaiming Your Body.* Berkeley, CA: North Atlantic Books.

Fallot, R. D., & Harris, M. (2009). *Creating Cultures of Trauma-Informed Care (CCTIC): A Self-Assessment and Planning Protocol.* www.researchgate.net/publication/272167009_Creating_Cultures_of_Trauma-Informed_Care_A_Self-Assessment_and_Planning_Protocol

Felitti, V. J., Anda, R. F., Nordenberg, D., Williamson, D. F. et al. (1998). Relationship of childhood abuse and household dysfunction to many of the leading causes of death in adults: The Adverse Childhood Experiences (ACE) Study. *American Journal of Preventive Medicine,* 14(4), 245–258. https://doi.org/10.1016/S0749-3797(98)00017-8

Frankl, V. (1962). *Man's Search for Meaning: An Introduction to Logotherapy.* Boston, MA: Beacon Press.

Frawley, D. (2010). *Mantra Yoga and Primal Sound: Secret Seed (Bija) Mantras.* Silver Lake, WI: Lotus Press.

Garner, G. (2016). *Medical Therapeutic Yoga: Biopsychosocial Rehabilitation and Wellness Care.* Edinburgh: Handspring Publishing.

Gersen, J. S. (2021). What if trigger warnings don't work? *The New Yorker,* September 28. www.newyorker.com/news/our-columnists/what-if-trigger-warnings-dont-work

Gilani, N. (2023). I teach yoga—its appropriation by the white wellness industry is a form of colonialism, but we can move on. *The Guardian,* January 3. www.theguardian.com/commentisfree/2023/jan/03/yoga-white-wellness-industry-21st-century-colonialism

Gill, N. (2019). The importance of trauma-informed design. Forbes. www.forbes.com/sites/forbesnonprofitcouncil/2019/12/09/the-importance-of-trauma-informed-design

Gluck, R. L., Hartzell, G. E., Dixon, H. D., Michopoulos, V. et al. (2021). Trauma exposure and stress-related disorders in a large, urban, predominantly African-American, female sample. *Archives of Women's Mental Health,* 24(6), 893–901.

Goddard, V. Z. (2021). The four immeasurables leave nothing untouched. Lion's Roar. www.lionsroar.com/the-four-immeasurables-leave-nothing-untouched

Grabovac, A. D., Lau, M. A., & Willett, B. R. (2011). Mechanisms of mindfulness: A Buddhist psychological model. *Mindfulness,* 2, 154–166.

Guidi, J., Lucente, M., Sonino, N., & Fava, G. A. (2020). Allostatic load and its impact on health: A systematic review. *Psychotherapy and Psychosomatics,* 90(1), 11–27.

Harris, G. (2021). *The Inspired Yoga Teacher: The Essential Guide to Creating Transformational Classes Your Students Will Love.* Eugene, OR: Luminary Press.

Harris, M., & Fallot, R. D. (2001). Envisioning a Trauma Informed Service System: A Vital Paradigm Shift. In M. Harris & R. D. Fallot (eds.) *Using Trauma Theory to Design Service Systems*. San Francisco, CA: JosseyBass.

International Association of Yoga Therapists (IAYT) (n.d.). Yoga therapy is... www.iayt.org/page/AboutLanding

Johnston, C. (1912). *The Yoga Sutras of Patanjali: The Book of the Spiritual Man—An Interpretation*. New York, NY: Kshetra Books.

Juruena, M. F., Eror, F., Cleare, A. J., & Young, A. H. (2020). The role of early life stress in HPA axis and anxiety. *Anxiety Disorders, 1191*, 141-153.

Karnes, A. (2023). Making yoga more inclusive: Language do's and don'ts for teachers. *Yoga International*. https://yogainternational.com/article/view/inclusive-yoga

Karoly, P. (1993). Mechanisms of self-regulation: A systems view. *Annual Review of Psychology, 44*(1), 23–52.

Keltner, D., Young, R. C., & Buswell, B. N. (1997). Appeasement in human emotion, social practice, and personality. *Aggressive Behavior, 23*(5), 359-374.

Koenen, K. C., Ratanatharathorn, A., Ng, L., McLaughlin, K. A. et al. (2017). Post-traumatic stress disorder in the World Mental Health Surveys. *Psychological Medicine, 47*, 2260-2274.

Kube, T., Berg, M., Kleim, B., & Herzog, P. (2020). Rethinking post-traumatic stress disorder: A predictive processing perspective. *Neuroscience & Biobehavioral Reviews, 113*, 448-460.

Lasater, J. H. (2021). *Teaching Yoga with Intention: The Essential Guide to Skillful Hands-on Assist and Verbal Communication*. Boulder, CO: Shambhala.

Lasater, J. H., & Lasater, I. K. (2022). *What We Say Matters: Practicing Nonviolent Communication* (revised edition). Boulder, CO: Shambhala.

Levine, P. (2010). *Healing Trauma: A Pioneering Program for Restoring the Wisdom of Your Body*. Boulder, CO: Sounds True.

Liasidou, A. (2022). Inclusive education as a trauma-responsive practice: Research-based considerations and implications. *International Journal of Inclusive Education*, 1-13. https://doi.org/10.1080/13603116.2022.2107720

Maharara, S., & Sabar, N. (2020). The concept of "OM": (with special reference to chāndogya upaniṣad). *International Journal of Sanskrit Research, 6*(3), 4-9.

McCain, A. (2023). 26 interesting yoga industry statistics: Yoga trends + review. Zippia. www.zippia.com/advice/yoga-industry-statistics

Menakem, R. (2017). *My Grandmother's Hands: Racialized Trauma and the Pathway to Mending Our Hearts and Bodies*. Las Vegas, NV: Central Recovery Press.

Mersky, J., Topitzes, J., Langlieb, J., & Dodge, K. A. (2021). Increasing mental health treatment access and equity through trauma-responsive care. *American Journal of Orthopsychiatry, 91*, 703-713.

Miller, R. (2022). *Yoga Nidra: The iRest Meditative Practice for Deep Relaxation and Healing*. Louisville, CO: Sounds True.

Morrison, K., & Dwarika, V. (2022). Trauma survivors' experiences of Kundalini yoga in fostering posttraumatic growth. *Journal of Child & Adolescent Trauma, 15*(3), 821-831.

Native Knowledge 360° (2023). Honoring original Indigenous inhabitants: Land acknowledgment. Smithsonian. https://americanindian.si.edu/nk360/informational/land-acknowledgment

Nummenmaa, L., Glerean, E., Hari, R., & Hietanen, J. K. (2014). Bodily maps of emotions. *Proceedings of the National Academy of Sciences, 111*(2), 646–651.

Ogden, P. (2021). *The Pocket Guide to Sensorimotor Psychotherapy in Context*. New York, NY: Guilford Press.

Oxford English Dictionary (2023). Intersectionality. www.oed.com/view/Entry/429843

Park, C. L., Riley, K. E., Bedesin, E., & Stewart, V. M. (2016). Why practice yoga? Practitioners' motivations for adopting and maintaining yoga practice. *Journal of Health Psychology, 21*(6), 887–896.

Parker, G. (2020). *Restorative Yoga for Ethnic and Race-Based Stress and Trauma*. London: Singing Dragon.

Porges, S. W. (1998). Love: An emergent property of the mammalian autonomic nervous system. *Psychoneuroendocrinology, 23*, 837–861.

Porges, S. W. (2017). *The Pocket Guide to the Polyvagal Theory: The Transformative Power of Feeling Safe*. New York, NY: W. W. Norton.

Porges, S. W. (2021). *Polyvagal Safety: Attachment, Communication, and Self-Regulation*. New York, NY: W. W. Norton.

Prabhavananda, S., & Isherwood, C. (2007). *How to Know God: The Yoga Aphorism of Patanjali*. Los Angeles, CA: Vedanta Press & Bookshop.

Ranganathan, S. (2008). *Patanjali's Yoga Sutra*. New York, NY: Penguin Books.

Ranganathan, S. (2023). *Yoga—Anticolonial Philosophy: An Action-Focused Guide to Practice*. London: Singing Dragon.

Riley, K. E., & Park, C. L. (2015). How does yoga reduce stress? A systematic review of mechanisms of change and guide to future inquiry. *Health Psychology Review, 9*(3), 379–396. https://doi.org/10.1080/17437199.2014.981778

Rosenberg, M. (2012). *Living Nonviolent Communication: Practical Tools to Connect and Communicate Skillfully in Every Situation*. Boulder, CO: Sounds True.

Ross, A., Friedmann, E., Bevans, M., & Thomas, S. (2012). Frequency of yoga practice predicts health: Results of a national survey of yoga practitioners. *Evidence-Based Complementary and Alternative Medicine*. https://doi.org/10.1155/2012/983258

Roze des Ordons, A. L., Ellaway, R. H., & Eppich, W. (2022). The many spaces of psychological safety in health professions education. *Medical Education, 56*(11), 1060–1063.

Satchidananda, S. S. (1985). *The Yoga Sutras of Patanjali*. Buckingham, VA: Integral Yoga Publications.

Schmidt, L. (2020). Incorporate LGBTQIIA+ inclusive language into your yoga class. Chopra. https://chopra.com/articles/incorporate-lgbtqia-inclusive-language-into-your-yoga-class

Scholte, S. (2023). History of the term "appeasement": A response to Bailey et al. (2023). *European Journal of Psychotraumatology, 14*(2), 2183005.

Schwartz, A. (2022). *Therapeutic Yoga for Trauma Recovery: Applying the Principles of the Polyvagal Theory for Self-Discovery, Embodied Healing, and Meaningful Change.* Eau Claire, WI: PESI Publishing.

Siegel, D. J. (2010). *The Mindful Therapist: A Clinician's Guide to Mindsight and Neural Integration.* New York, NY: W. W. Norton.

Sloan, D. M., & Marx, B. P. (2019). *Written Exposure Therapy for PTSD: A Brief Treatment Approach for Mental Health Professionals.* Washington, DC: American Psychological Association.

Souza, T. (2020). Responding to microaggressions in online learning environments during a pandemic. Academic Impressions. www.academicimpressions.com/blog/microaggressions-online-learning

Spence, J. (2021). *Trauma-Informed Yoga: A Toolbox for Therapists—47 Simple Practices to Calm, Balance, and Restore the Nervous System.* Eau Claire, WI: PESI Publishing.

Substance Abuse and Mental Health Services Administration (SAMHSA) (2014). *SAMHSA's Concept of Trauma and Guidance for a Trauma-Informed Approach.* SAMHSA's Trauma and Justice Strategic Initiative. https://ncsacw.samhsa.gov/userfiles/files/SAMHSA_Trauma.pdf

Sue, D. W., Capodilupo, C. M., Torino, G. C., Bucceri, J. M. et al. (2007). Racial microaggressions in everyday life: Implications for clinical practice. *American Psychologist, 62*(4), 271.

Taylor, J. (2021). Time to start activating your inner resources? Habits for Wellbeing. www.habitsforwellbeing.com/start-activating-your-inner-resources

Tedeschi, R. G., Cann, A., Taku, K., Senol-Durak, E., & Calhoun, L. G. (2017). The posttraumatic growth inventory: A revision integrating existential and spiritual change. *Journal of Traumatic Stress, 30,* 11–18.

Telles, S. (n.d.). How to do Bharadvaja's Twist in yoga. Everyday Yoga. www.everydayyoga.com/blogs/guides/how-to-do-bharadvaja_s-twist-in-yoga

Thompson-Hollands, J., Marx, B. P., & Sloan, D. M. (2019). Brief novel therapies for PTSD: Written exposure therapy. *Current Treatment Options in Psychiatry, 6*(2), 99–106.

van der Kolk, B. (2014). *The Body Keeps the Score: Brain, Mind, and Body in the Healing of Trauma.* New York, NY: Penguin Publishing.

Walker, P. (2013). *Complex PTSD: From Surviving to Thriving.* CreateSpace Independent Publishing Platform.

Weintraub, A. (2012). *Yoga Skills for Therapists: Effective Practices for Mood Management.* New York, NY: W. W. Norton.

Wu, X., Kaminga, A. C., Dai, W., Deng, J. et al. (2019). The prevalence of moderate-to-high posttraumatic growth: A systematic review and meta-analysis. *Journal of Affective Disorders, 243,* 408–415.

Yehuda, R., & Lehrner, A. (2018). Intergenerational transmission of trauma effects: Putative role of epigenetic mechanisms. *World Psychiatry, 17*(3), 243–257.

Yoga Alliance (2019). Inclusion: Working group paper. https://yastandards.com/wp-content/uploads/2022/05/YA-SRP-Inclusion-Working-Group-Paper-2019.pdf

REFERENCES

Yoga Alliance (2020a). Code of conduct. www.yogaalliance.org/Portals/0/policies/Code_Of_Conduct_Yoga_Alliance.pdf

Yoga Alliance (2020b). Scope of practice. www.yogaalliance.org/Portals/0/policies/Scope_Of_Practice_Yoga_Alliance.pdf

Zhang, N., Xiang, X., Zhou, S., Liu, H., He, Y., & Chen, J. (2022). Physical activity intervention and posttraumatic growth: A systematic review and meta-analysis. *Journal of Psychosomatic Research, 152*, 110675.

Index

accessibility 285
accountability 285
accountable spaces 274
acknowledgment and
    gratitude statement 35
action urges
    emotions experienced
        as 136
    journal prompts 133, 210
    riding wave of 209-10
    sensations associated with
        128, 132-3, 209-10
    and trauma memories
        18, 102, 103
activating and stimulating
    yoga practices 237-54
active engagement
    32, 43, 141, 161
adaptation
    poor 52, 58
    positive 52, 61
Adverse Childhood Events
    (ACEs) 39-40, 58
agency
    and active facilitation
        of choice 183
    'being with' supporting
        capacity for 203, 206
    in community
        agreements 279
    and consent 187
    in creating TIR space 285
    importance in yoga
        class 191, 195, 200
    and positive
        embodiment 99
    principle 16, 44
    as supported in trauma-
        sensitive yoga 42, 43
    as trauma-informed
        value 20, 173
ahimsa (non-harming) 93,
    146-7, 152, 162, 209, 278

alert engagement 114,
    118, 183, 275
allostatic load 52, 57-8
Alternate Nostril Breathing
    (Nadi Shodhanam)
    256, 258-9
Alternative Seated Twist Pose
    (Bharadvaja's Twist) 261
appeasement 21, 189-90
artful self-care 89-93
assisting
    case studies 185, 198-9
    different perspectives
        on 182, 185, 196-7
    guidelines 197-8
    hands-on 182, 196-7,
        200, 285
    including details in class
        descriptions 184-5
    journal prompts 185, 200
attuned teaching 215-16
attunement
    in artful self-care 89-90
    in co-regulation model 125
    in difficult
        circumstances 101
    in embodied self model 100
    as goal of TIR yoga
        teaching 131, 214, 217
    nature of 69
    with nervous system
        29-30, 111
    principle 22, 214
    with students 63
    teaching 22, 214
autonomic nervous system
    actions 114-15
    appeasement driven by 189
    branches of 111-12
    breath control providing
        access to 110
    PVT focusing on
        functions of 110-11

Baby Cobra Pose (Ardha
    Bhujangasana) 244
balancing and integrating
    yoga practices 255-72
Balancing Half Moon Pose
    (Ardha Chandrasana)
    269-70
Bee Breathing (Bhramari
    Pranayama) 250-1
being with
    breathing as powerful
        practice of 207-8
    eight limbs and
        grounding 208-9
    emotions, hand-over-
        heart practice 210
    going forward from 217
    the moment 256
    noticing, naming,
        and reorienting
        thoughts 212-14
    pendulation practice
        210-11
    poses 193, 221
    powerful role of 204
    principle 21, 206
    as quality of yoga
        practice 128, 133
    readiness for 286
    riding wave of sensation
        action urge 209-10
    sensations 128, 130, 132,
        147, 149, 206-7
    shift to working with 214
    teachers seeking to
        embody skills of 281
    as TIR yoga teaching
        practice 43, 203
    as transformational 21, 206
    what is there 205-6
Bellows Breath (Bhastrika
    Pranayama) 237-9
Belly Breathing 228

INDEX

Block Breathing 245
Boat Pose (*Navasana*) 249
body
  attunement with 131, 185
  'being with'/'working with' 192–3
  and choice 183, 187–8
  as dimension of self 99–101
  and dissociation 133–4
  felt sense of 158
  grounding 74, 213
  hyperarousal and reactivity 60
  immobilization in face of danger 183
  as internal factor of trauma 52
  journal prompts 90, 95, 137
  listening to 102–5, 208
  maps of emotion patterns of activation and deactivation 139
  nature of relationship with emotions and thoughts 205
  orienting 74–5
  in pendulation practice 210–11
  relation with brain 110, 112
  and sensations 127, 136–7, 140, 142, 207, 285
  and stress 57–8
  tensing 204
  trauma memories stored in 102
  union with mind 91, 145
body states
  as access point for self-regulation 117
  affecting feelings and thoughts 116–17
  attuning to students' 124–5
  embodiment of connection states 275–6
  relationship with thought and emotions 205
brave space 274
breath
  bringing awareness to 106
  connecting to movement 22, 85, 191, 219, 220
  connection states 275–6
  dysregulated 71, 72
  focus on slowing 69
  highlighting 22, 208
  journal prompt 220
  listening to 103
  and nervous system 110
  principle 22, 208, 219
  self-statement 213

and sensations 127, 129, 130, 132
Breathe-With practice 71, 74
breathing
  eight limbs and grounding 208–9
  journal prompt 208
  as powerful being-with practice 207–8
  Pranayama 33
  together, principle 17, 71
  understanding 85
Breath of Joy 249–50
breath rate 73, 119, 142, 158, 186
Bridge Pose (*Setu Bandhasana*) 246
burnout 17, 79–81, 95–6

calming and soothing yoga practices 71, 73, 215–16, 218–36
calmness
  activation levels 67
  dorsal vagal complex 113, 115
  parasympathetic nervous system 112
  on self-regulation scale 68–9, 142, 148, 215
  teacher training discussion questions 217
care *see* collective care; mindful self-care
case studies 34–5
  Catherine and de-escalation protocol 72
  Eric and physical touch 185
  Erica's teaching style 170–1
  George and state activation 141, 150
  Janice and mindful self-care 92
  Joanne and consent, touch, and confusion 198–9
  Joelle's teaching style 171
  Jose and physical touch 185
  Kara's effects of trauma 104–5
  professional boundaries 83–4
  Sam and sensations 129, 130
  Sandra and informed choice 187–8
  Sara's escalation 150–1
  Shannon and memories 140

Sky and state activation 141, 150
Sonja and Rachel preparing to teach 276
Cat Pose (*Bidalasana*) 262–3
Centers for Disease Control (CDC) 39–40, 62
central nervous system 57, 110–11
Chair Pose (*Utkatasana*) 241–2
challenge and growth
  body, feelings and thoughts 119
  as connection state 114, 116, 119, 161, 183, 276
  in cycle of rest and effort 123
  embodiment while teaching 276
  in growth zone 121, 122, 237
  polyvagal pathway 114
  polyvagal states 116
  on self-regulation scale 68, 142, 148, 215
Chanting Om 231
Child's Pose (*Balasana*) 59, 69, 185, 197, 209, 215, 223–4
choice
  active facilitation of 183
  authentic and real 125
  'being with' supporting capacity for 192, 206
  and body 183
  importance in yoga class 191, 195, 200
  informed 187–8
  journal prompts 184, 187, 190
  and non-violent communication 160, 161, 180
  ongoing 188
  and positive embodiment 99, 100
  practice of encouraging 183–4, 193–4
  principle 16, 21, 44, 183, 189, 193, 273
  in self-regulatory feedback loop 149
  self-statement 213
  and sensations 128–9, 130, 131, 151
  to stop, establishing 21, 189
  as supported in trauma-sensitive yoga 43, 44
  as TIR guiding value 65
  and TIR verbal cueing 190–1, 195

295

choice *cont.*
  and ventral vagal
    complex 113
  and 'working with' 214
  yoga teaching approaches
    emphasizing 42, 43
cleanliness 284
Cognitive Behavioral
  Therapy (CBT) 47–8
collective care 18, 92–3, 277
comfort zone 121–2,
  123, 126, 215
communication
  bi-directional, between
    brain and body 110, 112
  definition 155
  with Indigenous
    communities 179–80
  microaggression
    responses 177–8
  mindful and heartful
    listening 20, 156–9,
    167–8, 279
  mindful use of Sanskrit 179
  nonverbal 235, 275
  and positive
    embodiment 103
  privacy and discretion
    within 172–3
  sensations as 19,
    127–8, 135–6
  teacher training
    discussion questions
    143–4, 159, 180–1
  TIR language as
    inclusive 20, 174–6
  trigger and content
    warnings 171–2
  as TIR yoga teaching
    practice 43
  use of clarifying
    statements 186–7
  via body language 113
  via sensations 135–44, 147
  see also nonviolent
    communication
communities and trauma 54
communities of care 23, 277–8
community agreements
  23, 278–9
compassion fatigue
  17, 79–81, 95
complex trauma 42, 53–4
connection
  to body 74, 183, 192,
    213, 217, 281
  and communities
    of care 277–8
  competing with
    protection 106–7

to earth 69, 74
importance to humans 107
and microaggressions 177
mind-body 91
and nervous system 52, 58,
  106, 111, 113, 114–16, 203
to others 62, 124–5, 148, 167
practice 76–7
principle 19, 116
relationships with
  body, emotions,
  and thoughts 205
in self-regulatory feedback
  loop 149–50
and sensations 147
teacher training discussion
  questions 126, 152
and trauma 134
words facilitating 155–6, 161
as yoga concept 62, 200
connection states
  access points for
    self-regulation 117
  and action urges 132
  and active polyvagal
    pathways 114
  in community
    agreements 279
  down-regulating into 150
  exploring 115–16
  inside window of
    tolerance 121, 148, 215
  joy and play 257
  listening as core feature
    of 156, 158
  nonviolent communication
    supporting 160, 161, 167
  principles for practicing
    within 219
  qualities of 278
  as shared need 166
  and TIR yoga
    teaching 275–6
  understanding 118–19
consent 21, 186, 187–8,
  197–9, 200, 279
content warnings 20,
  30, 171–2, 180
contraindications 216, 225
co-regulation 109,
  124–5, 126, 231
Corpse Pose *see Savasana*
  (Corpse Pose)
Cow Pose (*Bitilasana*) 263
Crescent Lunge Pose
  (*Anjaneyasana*) 193, 248–9
Crocodile Pose 69, 244–5
cueing
  attuned 203
  benefits of 43

de-escalation protocol 76
frequency of 195
journal prompts 184, 195
non-responsiveness
  to 59, 60, 61
and sensitivity 104, 150
as student-centered
  practice 200
in teacher bios 185
teacher training discussion
  question 200
verbal 43, 188, 190–1,
  197, 221
ways of receiving 194

Dancer Pose
  (*Natarajasana*) 141
DBT *see* Dialectical Behavior
  Therapy (DBT) for PTSD
decor 284
de-escalation protocol
  17, 71, 72–6, 77
developmental trauma 53–4
Dialectical Behavior Therapy
  (DBT) for PTSD 46
discomfort 19, 122,
  131–2, 152, 177
discretion 20, 172–3, 180
dissociation 101, 113,
  120, 133–4, 196
dissociative symptoms 59, 61
dorsal dive 113
dorsal vagal areas 139
dorsal vagal complex
  (DVC) 112, 113–14, 115
down-regulating 17, 71,
  150, 151, 161, 232
Downward-Facing Dog Pose
  (*Adho Mukha Svanasana*)
  150–1, 242–3, 257

Eagle Pose (*Garudasana*)
  267–8
Easy Sitting Pose
  (*Sukhasana*) 209, 229
effort
  of body, honoring 106
  cycle of 123
  great, principle of 19, 123
  inside window of
    tolerance 121
  teacher training discussion
    question 126
  worthiness 75, 213,
    217, 219, 232, 252
eight limbs of yoga 33,
  41, 208–9, 278, 281
embodied presence 124–5

INDEX

embodied self-regulation
    and *ahimsa* and *satya* 146-7
    becoming competent at 147
    defining 145
    sensations as conceptual tool for 128-33
embodied states
    activation and sensations 141-3
    and active polyvagal pathways 114-15
    and connection states 275-6
    and nervous system self-regulation scale 142-3
    teacher training discussion question 126
    understanding 118-20
embodiment
    definition 101
    disembodiment 124
    embodied self model 100
    journal prompt 101
    of learning 32-4
    positive 86, 99-102, 103, 107, 108, 121, 125, 281
    teacher training discussion questions 108, 143-4
    and trauma 102
    of yoga 155-6
Emotional Freedom Technique (EFT) 46-7
emotions
    body maps of patterns of activation and deactivation 139
    and co-regulation 124-5
    hand-over-heart practice 210
    inner self-regulation for 62
    limbic system processing 118
    outside window of tolerance 124
    pendulation practice 210-11
    physiological aspects of 136-40, 149
    principle 22, 209
    relationship with 205
    as self-regulation access point 117
    and sensations 135, 136-40, 149, 151
    support for 46-8
    as trauma internal factor 52
    see also feelings
empowerment
    and choice 21, 193
    journal prompt 184

knowledge and awareness fostering 80
nonviolent communication supporting 160
statements of 194, 213
as trauma-informed value 40, 65, 78, 160, 173
in yoga 151, 273, 286
engagement 149
    see also active engagement; alert engagement
environment
    dissociation from 133-4
    exteroception 103, 106
    scanning for safety 105-6
environmental factors
    in adverse childhood events 39, 58
    and microaggressions 177
    as mindful self-care domain 89
escalation 69, 150-1
    see also de-escalation protocol
exercise
    excessive 283, 284
    as mindful self-care domain 88
explicit consent 187, 197
Exposure Therapy (ET) 48
external aspects of self 99-100, 101
external experiences 135, 136, 149
external factors 52, 53-5, 57
external information 103, 104, 285
exteroception
    awareness of outside 125
    awareness of sensations through 148
    body communicating via 102
    connection and protection processes arising from 147
    definition 103, 106
    in self-regulatory feedback loop 149
    and stimuli 127
    teacher training discussion question 108
    trauma affecting 104
exteroceptive awareness 136
exteroceptive skills 105
Eye Movement Desensitization Reprocessing (EMDR) therapy 47

fawning 21, 189-90
feelings
    body states and nervous system associations 116-17
    in connection states 118-19
    developing plans honoring 168
    and embodiment 99-100
    journal prompt 165
    of loving-kindness 121, 122
    and memory 140
    naming 164-5
    and nonviolent communication 161, 162, 164-5
    outside window of tolerance 148
    in protection states 119-20
    related to trauma exposure 60
    see also emotions
fight or flight
    body, feelings and thoughts 119
    interoceptive sensation 141
    mobilization in reaction to fear 116
    nonviolent communication 160-1, 164, 170
    outside window of tolerance 143, 237
    polyvagal blended states 116
    as protection state 115, 119, 150
    on self-regulation scale 68, 142, 148, 215
    in self-regulatory feedback loop 149
    and sensation action urge 209
    in sympathetic nervous system 111-12
    thoughts and cognitions 212
    ventral vagal complex not active during 113
five-pound weight guideline 67, 77
freeze
    automatic immobilization 104
    body, feelings and thoughts 120
    dorsal vagal complex activating 113-14
    immobilization in reaction to fear 116, 183

freeze *cont.*
  nonviolent
    communication 161
  outside window of
    tolerance 143
  polyvagal blended
    states 116
  as protection state 115,
    120
  on self-regulation scale
    68, 142, 148, 215
  in sympathetic nervous
    system 111–12
fun 90–1

Ground, Breathe, and
  Orient practice 69
grounding
  for 'being with' 208–9
  definition 74
  poses 239–40, 241, 260
  practice 66, 74
  self-statement 213
  as somatic skill 66
Grounding, Orienting,
  and Resourcing
  protocol 74–5, 76
growth
  active ventral vagal
    complex supporting
    112, 116
  discomfort from 19, 122
  personal 94
  positive 52, 58, 61
  posttraumatic 17, 61–2,
    63
  principle 19, 132
  and response 206
  self-determination as
    supportive to 44
  self-statements 213
  see also challenge
    and growth
growth zone 121, 122–3,
  126, 209, 215, 237

Half Plank Pose (*Chaturanga Dandasana*) 147
hand-over-heart practice 210
hearing 20, 103, 156,
  157, 158, 159, 162
heartful listening 20,
  158–9, 167–8, 279
Hero Pose (*Virasana*) 266
Horse Whinny 238
hydration 88
hyperarousal 59, 60
hypermobility 133–4, 219–20

immobilization
  dorsal vagal 111, 113, 114–15
  principle 21, 183
  in reaction to fear 116
  teacher training discussion
    question 200
  without fear 115
inclusion 174, 176, 285, 286
inclusive language
  20, 174–6, 181
Indigenous land
  acknowledgment 179–80
Indigenous peoples 175–6
informed choice/
  consent 187–8, 197
inner resources 17,
  65–6, 75, 213
insurance 216–17
intergenerational trauma 52–3
internal aspects of self 100–1
internal experiences
  42, 51, 149
internal factors 52–3, 57
Internal Family
  Systems (IFS) 47
internal information
  103, 104, 123, 285
International Association
  of Yoga Therapists
  (IAYT) 48, 82
interoception
  awareness of inside 125
  awareness of sensations
    through 148
  as challenging for trauma-
    affected people 102–3
  connection and
    protection processes
    arising from 147
  definition 102, 106
  orienting students
    towards 192–3
  in self-regulatory
    feedback loop 149
  and stimuli 127
  teacher training discussion
    question 108
  and TIR cueing 190–1
  trauma affecting 104
interoceptive awareness
  43, 136, 190–1, 192
interoceptive sensations
  141, 150

journaling 32

Knees to Chest Pose
  (*Apanasana*) 222

Lateral Spine Movement
  268–9
learning
  to be with sensations
    132, 134
  in community
    agreements 279
  discomfort from 19, 122
  by doing 29
  embodying 32–4
  in growth zone 121
  Sanskrit 179
  yoga mat as space for 204
Legs up the Wall Pose
  (*Viparita Karani*) 223
liability 197, 216–17
lighting 284
Lion's Breath (*Simhasana*)
  251–2
listening
  to body 102–5, 204, 208
  in community
    agreements 279
  mindful and heartful 20,
    156–9, 167–8, 279
  to needs of others
    162, 167–8
  to sensations 127, 128, 135
location and access 283
Locust Pose (*Salabhasana*)
  245–6
loving-kindness
  artful self-care 91–2
  in comfort zone 121
  in growth zone 122
  meditation 73
  meeting students
    with 20, 146
  and mindful listening 156
  as one of four
    immeasurables 66
  as quality of connection
    states 275, 278
  relationships with
    body, emotions,
    and thoughts 205
  as yoga concept 62, 107

medical advice 283
medical care 88
meditation
  case study 104–5
  creating foundation
    for joy 270–1
  daily practice 85
  examples of 216
  guided 253–4
  knowledge of
    consciousness from 273

INDEX

loving-kindness 73
mindful and collective care 93
  with an object 109
  orienting for safety 105-6
  practice plan 87
  simple heart-centered 234-5
memories
  emerging during training 67
  pendulation practice for 210-11
  physical, and sensations 135, 140-1, 149, 191
  recording 32
  trauma 18, 47, 48, 102, 103, 113, 140
merchandise 283
microaggressions 21, 177-8, 181
mindful awareness 42, 63, 67, 100, 155, 281
mindful listening 20, 156-7, 167-8, 279
mindfulness
  of communication content 171
  as mindful self-care domain 89
  as yoga concept 62
mindful self-care
  awareness, willingness, and work 80-1
  as collective care 18, 92
  as comprehensive 78
  creating and maintaining manageable teaching schedule 93
  daily 87-8
  as generous act 18, 91
  journal prompts 90, 91, 92, 95
  knowing and remembering your 'Why' 94-5
  mindful and collective care meditation 93
  as not selfish behavior 92
  ongoing professional development and supervision 94
  practice of embodying 89-93
  principles 17, 18, 79, 91, 92
  prioritizing 78-9
  seeking support 95
  teacher training discussion questions 95-6
  ten domains of 88-9
  see also self-care

mindful use of Sanskrit 179
mindful use of voice 185-6
mobilization
  autonomic nervous system actions 114-15
  principle 21, 183
  in reaction to fear 116
  sympathetic nervous system 111
  teacher training discussion question 200
  without fear 115
Modified Camel Pose (*Ustrasana*) 246-7
Modified Side Angle Pose (*Parsvakonasana*) 241
Mountain Pose (*Tadasana*) 69, 141, 209, 221-2
movement
  connecting breath to 22, 85, 191, 219, 220
  deceptive 237-8
  hemispheres of brain as responsible for coordination of 255
music 233-4, 283

Nasal Breathing 230, 256
needs
  developing plan to honor 168
  expressing own 165-6
  of others, listening to and sensing 167-8
nemo dat quod non habet 18, 84
nervous system
  activating and stimulating practices 237-54
  assessing safety and threat 18, 103, 104
  balancing and integrating practices 255-71
  being with 205
  breath as most direct access to 207
  breathing helping dysregulated 17, 71
  connection and protection as competing drives of 106-8
  connection and protection functions 58
  embodied awareness of 85
  impact of trauma 52, 54, 57-8, 116
  journal prompts 53, 276
  mindful awareness of 67
  recommended practices 86

relationship with yoga 29
science and theory 110-20
self-regulation scale 68-9, 142, 148
soothing and calming practices 69, 73, 218-35
teacher training discussion questions 108, 235-6, 254, 272
TIR yoga teachers' relationship with 275-6
trauma defined by impact of event on 16, 51
see also autonomic nervous system; central nervous system; parasympathetic nervous system; peripheral nervous system; polyvagal theory (PVT); sympathetic nervous system
neuroception
  assessing safety and threat 103-4, 148, 151
  freeze response 120
  listening to body 102
  principle 18, 104
  in self-regulatory feedback loop 149
  and stimuli 127
  teacher training discussion question 108
  trauma affecting 104
nonviolent communication
  beginning with awareness 160
  in community agreements 279
  definition 161
  developing plan honoring feeling and needs 168
  expressing needs 165-6
  fusing ahimsa and satya 161
  journal prompts 163, 165, 166, 167
  listening to and sensing needs of others 167-8
  making observations 162-3
  making request 166-7
  and microaggressions 177-8
  naming feelings 164-5
  principle 20, 161
  supportive functions 160-1
  teacher training discussion questions 169
  as ventral vagal practice 161

299

nutrition 88
nutritional advice 283

observation
  cueing 195
  inner 278
  journal prompt 163
  as nonviolent
    communication
    step 162-3
  responding to
    microaggressions 178
  and sensations 133
  of students 204, 208
  teacher training discussion
    question 181
Observe, Think, Feel,
  and Desire 178
Ocean-Sounding Breathing
  (Ujjayi Pranayama) 270
ongoing consent 188, 198
opting out 191, 285
options 21, 44, 190-1,
  193-4, 285
orienting
  for safety 18, 105-6
  techniques 69, 74-5
  toward inner
    experiences 42
  toward interoception
    190-1, 192-3
  toward protection
    52, 57, 108
  see also reorienting

parasympathetic
  nervous system 111,
    112, 114, 231, 270
Patanjali 84, 145, 278
PAUSE
  being with offering 205
  on the edge 121
  journal prompt 71
  practicing 124, 142,
    162, 206, 219
  principle 17, 70
  in self-regulatory
    feedback loop 149
  teacher training discussion
    question 77
  three step process 70
  as trauma-informed
    practice 70
  when down-regulating 150
pendulation practice 210-11
peripheral nervous
  system 110-11
permission 216-17

personal practice see practice;
  scope of practice
physical activities 86, 88
physical aspects of memory
  135, 140-1, 149, 191
physical care 88
physical health 41, 110, 177
physical space 283
physical therapy 134,
  150, 282, 283
physiological aspects of
  emotions 136-40, 149
physiological experiences 136
Pigeon Pose on the Mat 264-5
Pigeon Pose variations 263-5
Plank Pose (Kumbhakasana)
  247
polyvagal theory (PVT)
  blended states 116
  creator of 103
  focus of 111
  further resources 126
  introduction 109
  nature of 110
  pathways of 114-15
  principle 18, 110
  in relation to nervous
    system 111, 237
  teacher training discussion
    question 126
Porges, S. 9, 103, 106, 107,
  109, 110, 112-13, 126, 207
positive embodiment see
  embodiment: positive
posttraumatic growth
  17, 61-2, 63
posttraumatic stress
  disorder (PTSD)
  and breathing-only
    interventions 208-9
  DBT for 46
  and dissociative
    symptoms 59, 61
  prevalence 62-3
  trauma-sensitive yoga 42
  WET for 48
potentially traumatizing
  events (PTEs) 51, 52,
    54, 56-7, 58-9, 63
practice
  associated with mindful
    self-care 88-9
  frequency of 85-6
  importance of 18, 33-4, 85
  journal prompt 86
  list of TIR 24-7
  orienting for safety
    prior to 105
  in pain-free range of
    motion 22, 218

personal, developing and
  maintaining 84-5, 87
plan 87
principle 18, 85
universal 43, 44, 49
see also scope of practice
privacy 20, 172-3,
  180, 279, 282
professional boundaries
  in creating TIR space 284
  journal prompt 84
  practice of keeping 82-4
  principle 18, 82
professional development
  78, 82, 94, 96
props 220, 221, 232-4, 236, 282
protection
  competing with
    connection 106-7
  fear as primary feeling
    associated with 107-8
  importance to survival
    107, 165
  and nervous system 51, 52,
    57, 58, 106, 107-8, 111
  principle 19, 116
  relationships with
    body, emotions,
    and thoughts 205
  and sensations 147, 150, 271
  and trauma 108
protection states
  access points for
    self-regulation 117
  and action urges 132, 209
  and active polyvagal
    pathways 115
  exploring 115-16
  nonviolent communication
    160, 161
  outside window of
    tolerance 121, 148, 215
  power of words 155, 161
  regularly escalating
    into 150
  teacher training discussion
    questions 126, 152
  and TIR yoga teaching 170
  and trauma 212-13
  understanding 119-20
Pyramid Pose
  (Parsvottanasana)
  215, 225-6

range of motion 22,
  133, 218, 219-20
Ratio Breathing 231, 256
reactivity 51, 59, 60, 148
Reclining Bound Angle

INDEX

Pose (*Supta Baddha Konasana*) 225
Reclining Pigeon Pose 265
Reclining Spinal Twist Pose (*Supta Matsyendrasana*) 262
recognizing
  in de-escalation protocol 17, 71, 72, 76
  identities 179–80, 274, 279
  sensations 128, 142
re-experiencing 59, 172
referring
  in de-escalation protocol 17, 43, 71, 75–6
  to identities 175, 176
relationships
  with body, emotions, and thoughts 205
  connection supporting 107
  as mindful self-care domain 89, 91
  and nonviolent communication 166–7, 168
  and sensations 128–9
reorienting
  journal prompt 214
  self-statements 213
  thoughts 22, 211, 212–13
resourcing 75, 76
responsiveness 59, 90, 124, 214
rest
  cycle of 123
  great, principle of 19, 123
  as mindful self-care domain 88
  teacher training discussion question 126
rest, restoration, and recovery
  body, feelings and thoughts 118
  in comfort zone 121
  as connection state 114, 116, 118, 183
  inside window of tolerance 121
  polyvagal blended states 116
Reverse Table Top Pose (*Ardha Purvottanasana*) 243–4
Reverse Warrior Pose (*Viparita Virabhadrasana*) 240

safety
  in community agreements 279

considerations 45–9
and co-regulation 125
in creating TIR space 282
feeling unsafe 19
and nervous system 51, 58, 103–4, 106, 107–8, 111, 112, 113, 185–6
orienting for 18, 105–6
safe and uncomfortable principle 19, 122
safe space 22, 274
self-statement 213
and sensations 19, 130–1, 134, 148, 206
as shared need 165–6
as TIR principle 16, 45
trauma affecting sense of 54
as trauma-informed value 40, 78, 273, 279
Sandbag Breathing 228
Sanskrit 179, 221, 231, 235, 281
satya (truth) 93, 101, 146–7, 152, 162, 209, 278
Savasana (Corpse Pose) 232–4
  aka lying down pose 118
  and assists 198, 199
  in case studies 140, 199
  confusion with meditation 234
  as deeply relaxing 118
  experience of feeling-sensations 137
  journal prompts 141, 234
  missing, as trauma presentation in class 59, 61
  sensation action urge example 209–10
  teacher training discussion question 235
scope of practice 17, 81–3, 96
Seated Pigeon Pose (*Kapotasana*) 264
Seated Twist Pose (*Parivrtta Sukhasana*) 260–1
seeing 20, 117–20, 156, 157, 158, 159
self-awareness
  cues orienting students towards 42
  as mindful self-care domain 89
  and nonviolent communication 160–1
  teaching 203–17
  as yoga concept 62
self-care *see* mindful self-care
self-compassion 62, 88
self-determination

and active facilitation of choice 183
'being with' supporting capacity for 203, 206
in community agreements 279
and consent 187
importance in yoga class 191, 200
self-statement 213
as shared need 165
as supported in trauma-sensitive yoga 42
as supportive to student growth 44
trauma affecting 54
as trauma-informed value 20, 173
self-regulation
  access points for 117
  access to 148
  assessing 67
  and connection state 275
  and co-regulation 124–5
  goal of TIR techniques 105
  ground, breathe, and orient for 69
  interoception helping 102
  responsibility for 161
  self-statements 213
  and sensations 147–51
  taking time for 22
  teacher training discussion questions 126, 152
  for TIR yoga teachers, principle 22, 275
  yoga as 43
  as yoga concept 62
  see also embodied self-regulation
self-regulation scale
  and attuned teaching 215
  in comfort zone 121
  in connection mode 107
  in cycle of rest and effort 123
  enhanced 148, 215
  journal prompts 68, 69, 71
  nervous system 68, 142, 255
  and PAUSE 70–1
  practice 68–9
  principle 17, 68
  states of embodiment 114–15, 142–3
  teacher training discussion questions 77, 108, 152
self-regulatory feedback loop 149, 150, 152
self-soothing 88
self-statements 213–14

301

sensations
  action urges accompanying 209-10
  being with 21, 206-7
  clarifying 186-7
  as communication 19, 127-8, 135-6
  communication via 135-44, 147
  definition 127
  detection of 149
  as experiences 19, 135, 136-40, 143-4
  and exteroception 106
  hand-over-heart practice 210
  hypermobility and dissociation 133-4
  and interoception 102-3, 141, 148, 192-3
  journal prompts 95, 132, 137, 140, 143, 211
  noticing vs. sensation seeking 133
  pendulation practice 210-11
  and safety 19, 130-1, 134, 148, 206
  and satya 147
  and self-regulation 148-51
  and self-regulatory feedback loop 149, 150
  sources of 149
  teacher training discussion questions 134, 136, 143-4
  teaching to notice 22, 214
  and tone of sensation, factors affecting 131
  traits of 128-33
  and trauma-informed cueing 191
  and trauma memories 18, 102
sensitivity
  affecting interoception, exteroception, and neuroception 104-5
  decreased 104
  increased 51, 104
Shaking 252
shutdown
  attuning to 203
  body, feelings and thoughts 120
  dorsal vagal complex activating 113-14
  hyperarousal and reactivity 60

immobilization in reaction to fear 116, 183
interoceptive sensations 141
journal prompt 61
nonviolent communication 160, 161, 170
outside window of tolerance 121, 124, 143
polyvagal blended states 116
as protection state 115, 120, 170
on self-regulation scale 215
in self-regulatory feedback loop 149
thoughts and cognitions 212
Side Plank Pose (*Vasisthasana*) 150-1, 248
Sighing Breath 228-9
social and mental health support 45-6
social engagement system 107, 111, 113, 124-5
somatic nervous system 110-11
soul wound 53
Spinal Extension Pose 259
spiritual practice
  as mindful self-care domain 89
  yoga as 81, 280
spiritual speech 163
stabilizing 17, 71, 72-4, 76
Staff Pose (*Dandasana*) 265-6
Stair-Step Breathing (*Viloma 1*) 230
Standing Forward Fold (*Uttanasana*) 215, 224-5, 257
Standing Squat Pose (*Utkata Konasana*) 252-3
state activation
  in-the-moment 135
  in self-regulatory feedback loop 149
  sensations communicating 141-3
  shaping thoughts 22, 211
  teacher training discussion questions 143, 152
statements
  aligned with nonviolent communication 165
  clarifying, use in yoga classes 186-7
  contrasting supportive and harmful 194
  "I" 178, 279

journal prompts 165, 187, 214
judgment-filled 163
reorienting self-statements 213-14
unhelpful 164-5
stopping
  practice of offering choice 189
  principle of choice 21, 189
stress
  blocking access to joy 257
  and dissociation 133-4
  journal prompt 58
  and nervous system 51, 57-8, 109, 113, 116, 189, 237
  and scope of practice 81-2
  and trauma 52, 53, 116
  and triggers 172
  and window of tolerance 121
  yoga working to lessen impact of 40-1
sympathetic nervous system 111-12, 113, 114-16, 155, 237, 238, 254
systemic trauma 54

taking action 90
teachers
  biographies 184-5
  in creating TIR space 281
  teaching within permitted scope 81-2
  trauma-informed, addressing microaggressions 21, 177-8
teaching schedules 93
teaching yoga *see* trauma-informed and responsive (TIR) yoga teaching
thoughts
  as access point for self-regulation 117
  becoming mirrors of reactive state 148
  in connection state 118-19
  in embodied self model 100
  as internal factor of trauma 52
  journal prompts 122, 123, 124, 214
  and mindfulness 89
  nature of relationships with body and emotions 205-6

INDEX

negative, as symptom of PTSD 59
  in nonviolent communication 161
  noting, naming, and reorienting 212–14
  in protection state 119–20, 212–13
  sensation-related, in yoga poses 129–30
  as symptom of trauma 60
  TF-CBT for 47
  trauma and state activation shaping 22, 211
touch
  case study 198–9
  different perspectives on 185
  exteroception 103, 136
  giving careful consideration to 196–8
  guidelines 197–8
  journal prompts 185, 200
  teacher training discussion question 200
trauma
  avoiding reminders 59
  blocking access to joy 257
  causes and effects of 52
  definition 54
  depiction of causes and effects 53
  as disintegrating force 102
  effects of 56–62
  event/exposure factors 55–6
  external factors 53–5
  and impact 16, 51, 52
  internal factors 52–3
  journal prompts 58, 61
  nature of 50–1
  nervous system and yoga 110–20
  prevalence 44–5, 62–3
  and protection state thoughts 212–13
  and sensations 127, 131
  shaping thoughts 22, 211
  symptomatology, factors contributing to risk of 55–6
  teacher training discussion questions 63–4
  TIR as not a treatment for 43–4
  as universal 17, 63
Trauma Center Trauma-Sensitive Yoga (TCTSY) 42
trauma exposure
  factors contributing to risk of trauma symptomatology 55–6
  journal prompt 56
  prevalence of 62–3
  symptoms related to 59–61
  as varying 16, 55, 56–7
Trauma-Focused Cognitive Behavioral Therapy (TF-CBT) 47–8
trauma-focused (TF) work 28
trauma-informed and responsive (TIR) care 39–40
trauma-informed and responsive (TIR) communication *see* communication; nonviolent communication
trauma-informed and responsive (TIR) methods 29, 42–5, 48–9
trauma-informed and responsive (TIR) spaces
  changing 274–5
  creating 280–6
  cultivating 273–4
  journal prompt 286
  need for more 274
  teacher training discussion questions 286
  as unique 23, 280
trauma-informed and responsive (TIR) yoga teaching
  beginning with choice and agency 16, 44
  communities of care 23, 277–8
  community agreements 23, 278–9
  and connection states 275–6
  and co-regulation 124–5
  defining 42–3
  evolution of 40–1
  guiding values 65
  integrating joy and play in 257
  journal prompts 276, 277
  list of practices 24–7
  list of principles 16–23
  as not treatment for trauma 43–4
  personal practice as foundation of 18, 85
  preparing to teach 276–7
  sensations as pertinent to 127, 134, 135
  teacher training discussion questions 49, 143–4
  terminology of 41–5
  trauma-informed practice 70–1
  trauma-informed values/ principles 40, 65, 78, 173
  trauma-informed yoga teaching practices 43
  trauma memories 18, 47, 48, 102, 103, 113, 140
  trauma-related disorder 52, 58–9
  trauma-responsive yoga teaching practices 43
  trauma-sensitive yoga 42, 196
Tree Pose (*Vrksasana*) 255, 256, 257–8
Triangle Pose (*Trikonasana*) 227–8
triggers 150, 171–2

union 91, 145
Upward-Facing Dog Pose (*Urdhva Mukha Svanasana*) 243

ventral vagal areas 138, 139
ventral vagal complex (VVC) 112–13, 115, 237, 255
ventral vagal state *see* connection states
verbal cueing 43, 188, 190–1, 197, 221
vicarious trauma 54
voice
  access to 99
  in community agreements 279
  connection states 275–6
  embodiment of connection states while teaching 275–6
  journal prompts 186, 277
  Lion's Breath for 251–2
  mindful use of 185–6
  as trauma-informed principle 40, 273

Warrior Pose 1 (*Virabhadrasana 1*) 129, 226–7
Warrior Pose 2 (*Virabhadrasana 2*) 130, 239–40
Warrior Pose 3 (*Virabhadrasana 3*) 260

WET *see* Written Exposure
    Therapy (WET)
window of tolerance
    definition 121
    edge of 121, 123–4
    expanding 209
    inside 121–3, 148, 215, 255
    journal prompt 124
    outside 121, 124, 143,
        148, 215, 237
    of students in yoga class
        131
    teacher training discussion
        question 126
    usefulness 109
working with
    discomfort 19, 132
    emotions 151
    journal prompt 214
    pain-free range of
        motion 219
    poses 193, 221, 257
    readiness for 286
    sensations 128, 130,
        132, 147, 149
    teachers seeking to
        embody skills of 281
    as TIR yoga teaching
        practice 43, 203
    what is here 205, 214
Written Exposure
    Therapy (WET) 48

yoga
    activating and stimulating
        practices 237–54
    balancing and integrating
        practices 255–72
    as both trigger and
        tool for working
        with trauma 28
    in creating TIR space 281
    eight limbs 33, 41,
        208–9, 278, 281
    as embodied practice 99
    endings for
        transformation 286
    essence as attuned,
        compassionate
        connection 200
    as experience of positive
        embodiment in
        which we abide in
        our true nature 101
    foundational model for 91
    helping to develop
        inner resources 66
    honoring roots of 33
    as inherently trauma-
        informed and
        responsive 146
    as intentional, self-
        determined practice
        of mobilizing and
        immobilizing the
        body 21, 183
    in learning by doing
        category 29
    nervous system and
        trauma 110–20
    number of people
        practicing 41
    as offering guidance 23, 278
    as personal 16, 41
    and post-traumatic
        growth 61–2
    role of touch 197
    Sanskrit as language of 179
    soothing and calming
        practices 218–35
    as soulful practice 78
    as spiritual and secular
        practice 23, 280
    as stilling of mind to find
        unity within 205
    studying 33
    trauma-sensitive 42, 196
    two truths in relation
        to trauma 28
    working to reduce impact
        of stress 40–1
    see also trauma-informed
        and responsive (TIR)
        yoga teaching
Yoga Alliance 33, 41, 81–2,
    94, 174, 175, 197–8
yoga class
    detailed descriptions
        184–5
    goal of, in yoga sutra 145
    highlighting breath
        in 22, 207–8
    inviting students
        into 191–2
    journal prompts 61, 200
    post-traumatic growth
        presentation in 62
    as practice of moving in
        and out of comfort
        and growth zones 123
    as process for tying strands
        of mind together 145
    seeing body states
        in 117–20
    as sensational 128
    teacher training discussion
        questions 63–4, 77
    touch, consent and
        confusion 198–200
    trauma symptoms
        presentation in 59–61
    using clarifying statements
        early in 186–7
yoga mat 30, 45, 204
yoga students
    asking for help 76–7
    co-regulation 124–5
    engaging in appeasement
        21, 189–90
    inviting into yoga asana
        or practice 191–2
    meeting where they
        are 20, 146
    orienting toward
        interoception 192–3
Yoga Therapy 48, 82